Local Government Actions to Prevent Childhood Obesity

Committee on Childhood Obesity Prevention Actions for Local Governments

Food and Nutrition Board
Board on Children, Youth, and Families
Board on Population Health and Public Health Practice
Transportation Research Board

Lynn Parker, Annina Catherine Burns, and Eduardo Sanchez, *Editors*

INSTITUTE OF MEDICINE *AND*
NATIONAL RESEARCH COUNCIL
OF THE NATIONAL ACADEMIES

THE NATIONAL ACADEMIES PRESS
Washington, D.C.
www.nap.edu

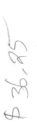

THE NATIONAL ACADEMIES PRESS   500 Fifth Street, N.W.   Washington, DC 20001

NOTICE: The project that is the subject of this report was approved by the Governing Board of the National Research Council, whose members are drawn from the councils of the National Academy of Sciences, the National Academy of Engineering, and the Institute of Medicine. The members of the committee responsible for the report were chosen for their special competences and with regard for appropriate balance.

This study was supported by Grant No. 61747 between the National Academy of Sciences and The Robert Wood Johnson Foundation and Contract No. 200-2005-13434, Task Order 13, between the National Academy of Sciences and the Centers for Disease Control and Prevention. Any opinions, findings, conclusions, or recommendations expressed in this publication are those of the author(s) and do not necessarily reflect the view of the organizations or agencies that provided support for this project.

Library of Congress Cataloging-in-Publication Data

Institute of Medicine (U.S.). Committee on Childhood Obesity Prevention Actions for Local Governments.
  Local government actions to prevent childhood obesity / Committee on Childhood Obesity Prevention Actions for Local Governments, Food and Nutrition Board . . . [et al.] ; Lynn Parker, Annina Catherine Burns, and Eduardo Sanchez, editors.
      p. ; cm.
  Includes bibliographical references.
  ISBN 978-0-309-13927-4 (pbk.) — ISBN 978-0-309-13928-1 (pdf) 1. Obesity in children—United States. I. Parker, Lynn. II. Burns, Annina Catherine. III. Sanchez, Eduardo (Eduardo J.) IV. Title.
  [DNLM: 1. Obesity—prevention & control—United States. 2. Child—United States. 3. Government Programs—United States. 4. Health Promotion—organization & administration—United States. 5. Local Government—United States. WD 210 I602L 2009]
  RJ399.C6I573 2009
  618.92′398—dc22

                                                            2009044336

Additional copies of this report are available from the National Academies Press, 500 Fifth Street, N.W., Lockbox 285, Washington, DC 20055; (800) 624-6242 or (202) 334-3313 (in the Washington metropolitan area); Internet, http://www.nap.edu.

For more information about the Institute of Medicine, visit the IOM home page at: **www.iom.edu.**

The serpent has been a symbol of long life, healing, and knowledge among almost all cultures and religions since the beginning of recorded history. The serpent adopted as a logotype by the Institute of Medicine is a relief carving from ancient Greece, now held by the Staatliche Museen in Berlin.

Suggested citation: IOM (Institute of Medicine) and National Research Council. 2009. *Local Government Actions to Prevent Childhood Obesity.* Washington, DC: The National Academies Press.

"Knowing is not enough; we must apply.
Willing is not enough; we must do."
—Goethe

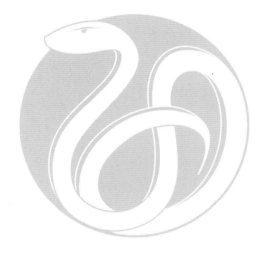

INSTITUTE OF MEDICINE
OF THE NATIONAL ACADEMIES

Advising the Nation. Improving Health.

THE NATIONAL ACADEMIES
Advisers to the Nation on Science, Engineering, and Medicine

The **National Academy of Sciences** is a private, nonprofit, self-perpetuating society of distinguished scholars engaged in scientific and engineering research, dedicated to the furtherance of science and technology and to their use for the general welfare. Upon the authority of the charter granted to it by the Congress in 1863, the Academy has a mandate that requires it to advise the federal government on scientific and technical matters. Dr. Ralph J. Cicerone is president of the National Academy of Sciences.

The **National Academy of Engineering** was established in 1964, under the charter of the National Academy of Sciences, as a parallel organization of outstanding engineers. It is autonomous in its administration and in the selection of its members, sharing with the National Academy of Sciences the responsibility for advising the federal government. The National Academy of Engineering also sponsors engineering programs aimed at meeting national needs, encourages education and research, and recognizes the superior achievements of engineers. Dr. Charles M. Vest is president of the National Academy of Engineering.

The **Institute of Medicine** was established in 1970 by the National Academy of Sciences to secure the services of eminent members of appropriate professions in the examination of policy matters pertaining to the health of the public. The Institute acts under the responsibility given to the National Academy of Sciences by its congressional charter to be an adviser to the federal government and, upon its own initiative, to identify issues of medical care, research, and education. Dr. Harvey V. Fineberg is president of the Institute of Medicine.

The **National Research Council** was organized by the National Academy of Sciences in 1916 to associate the broad community of science and technology with the Academy's purposes of furthering knowledge and advising the federal government. Functioning in accordance with general policies determined by the Academy, the Council has become the principal operating agency of both the National Academy of Sciences and the National Academy of Engineering in providing services to the government, the public, and the scientific and engineering communities. The Council is administered jointly by both Academies and the Institute of Medicine. Dr. Ralph J. Cicerone and Dr. Charles M. Vest are chair and vice chair, respectively, of the National Research Council.

www.national-academies.org

COMMITTEE ON CHILDHOOD OBESITY PREVENTION ACTIONS FOR LOCAL GOVERNMENTS

EDUARDO J. SANCHEZ (*Chair*), Vice President and Chief Medical Officer, Blue Cross and Blue Shield of Texas, Richardson

PEGGY BELTRONE, Commissioner, Cascade County Commission, Great Falls, MT

LAURA K. BRENNAN, President and CEO, Transtria, LLC, St. Louis, MO

JOSEPH A. CURTATONE, Mayor, City of Somerville, Somerville, MA

ERIC A. FINKELSTEIN, RTI International, Research Triangle Park, NC

TRACY FOX, President, Food, Nutrition, and Policy Consultants, Washington, DC

SUSAN L. HANDY, Professor in the Department of Environmental Science and Policy, University of California at Davis

JAMES KRIEGER, Chief of the Chronic Disease and Injury Prevention Section, Public Health–Seattle and King County, Seattle, WA

DONALD DIEGO ROSE, Associate Professor, Community Health Sciences, Tulane University School of Public Health and Tropical Medicine, New Orleans, LA

MARY T. STORY, Professor, Division of Epidemiology and Community Health, University of Minnesota School of Public Health, Minneapolis

ADEWALE TROUTMAN, Director, Louisville Metro Department of Public Health and Wellness, Louisville, KY

ANTRONETTE K. (TONI) YANCEY, Professor of Health Services, University of California at Los Angeles School of Public Health

PAUL ZYKOFSKY, Director, Land Use/Transportation Programs, Local Government Commission, Sacramento, CA

Study Staff

LYNN PARKER, Study Director

ANNINA CATHERINE BURNS, Program Officer

CATHARYN T. LIVERMAN, Scholar

NICOLE FERRING, Research Associate

MATTHEW B. SPEAR, Senior Program Assistant

ANTON L. BANDY, Financial Associate

GERALDINE KENNEDO, Administrative Assistant

LINDA D. MEYERS, Director, Food and Nutrition Board

Reviewers

This report has been reviewed in draft form by individuals chosen for their diverse perspectives and technical expertise, in accordance with procedures approved by the National Research Council's Report Review Committee. The purpose of this independent review is to provide candid and critical comments that will assist the institution in making its published report as sound as possible and to ensure that the report meets institutional standards for objectivity, evidence, and responsiveness to the study charge. The review comments and draft manuscript remain confidential to protect the integrity of the deliberative process. We wish to thank the following individuals for their review of this report:

DON BISHOP, Minnesota Department of Health, St. Paul, MN

KELLY BROWNELL, Rudd Center for Food Policy and Obesity, Yale University, New Haven, CT

MICHAEL CALDWELL, Health Officer, Dutchess County, NY

EVE HIGGINBOTHAM, Morehouse School of Medicine, Atlanta, GA

ALLISON KARPYN, Director of Research and Evaluation, The Food Trust, Philadelphia, PA

GEORGE LEVENTHAL, Councilmember, Montgomery County Council, MD

MALISA McCREEDY, Families, Parks and Recreation Department, City of Orlando, FL

MIRIAM NELSON, Tufts University, Boston, MA

SARAH SAMUELS, President, Samuels and Associates, Oakland, CA

WILL WYNN, Mayor, Austin, TX (Ret.)

Although the reviewers listed above have provided many constructive comments and suggestions, they were not asked to endorse the conclusions or recommendations nor did they see the final draft of the report before its release. The review of this report was overseen by **HUGH TILSON,** University of North Carolina, and **JOHANNA DWYER,** Tufts University Schools of Medicine and Nutrition. Appointed by the National Research Council and Institute of Medicine, they were responsible for making certain that an independent examination of this report was carried out in accordance with institutional procedures and that all review comments were carefully considered. Responsibility for the final content of this report rests entirely with the authoring committee and the institution.

Preface

This report is the first in a series of publications dedicated to providing brief, succinct information on childhood obesity prevention specifically for policy makers. Funded by The Robert Wood Johnson Foundation and the Centers for Disease Control and Prevention, the report focuses on one of the major recommendations in two previous Institute of Medicine (IOM) reports on obesity (*Preventing Childhood Obesity: Health in the Balance* and *Progress in Preventing Childhood Obesity: How Do We Measure Up?*) regarding the vital role of local governments in helping to prevent childhood obesity.

When people look back 50 years from now, childhood obesity may well stand out as the most important public health issue of our time. The prevalence of childhood obesity has tripled in just three decades, contributing to the ever more frequent appearance in children and youth of what were once chronic diseases and conditions usually associated with adulthood—"adult-onset" diabetes, high blood pressure, and high cholesterol. There is no more sobering thought than the growing consensus that the life expectancy of many of today's children will be less than their parents' because of the impact of early and continuing obesity on their health.

The good news is that much can and is being done in all sectors of our society to reverse this dangerous trend and its sad and costly consequences. This report focuses on the food and physical activity environments in which children live, study, and play, and recommends local government actions that have the potential to improve these environments by making healthy eating and optimum physical activity possible and easy for all children. The report also highlights the value of understanding the local context in which decisions are made on childhood obesity prevention efforts; the importance of paying particular attention to community conditions that result in unequal access to opportunities for healthy foods and physical activity, and therefore contribute to health disparities; and the need for evaluation of local childhood obesity prevention actions to learn more about what works. It is our hope that the report will find its way to local government officials and community members who can put what we have learned to good use in their efforts to improve the present and future health of their children and their communities.

I want to express my sincere appreciation and thanks to the committee members for their deep commitment to our task and the countless volunteer hours they contributed to this study and the development of the report. I also want to thank our excellent and thought-provoking workshop speakers, Marice Ashe, Matthew Longjohn, and Gerardo Mouet, for the insight and perspectives they brought to bear regarding local government initiatives on childhood obesity prevention. In addition, many thanks to Rona Briere for her valuable copyediting. Finally, I want to express my gratitude to the dedicated IOM staff who worked with the committee on this project: Lynn Parker, Study Director; Annina Burns, Program Officer; Nicole Ferring, Research Associate; Matthew Spear, Senior Program Assistant; Cathy Liverman, Scholar; and Linda Meyers, Food and Nutrition Board Director. I also wish to thank their IOM and National Research Council collaborators: Rosemary Chalk, Director of the Board on Children, Youth, and Families; Nancy Humphrey, Senior Program Officer in the Studies and Special Program Division of the Transportation Research Board; and Rose Marie Martinez, Director of the Board on Population Health and Public Health Practice.

Eduardo Sanchez, *Chair*
Committee on Childhood Obesity Prevention Actions
for Local Governments

Contents

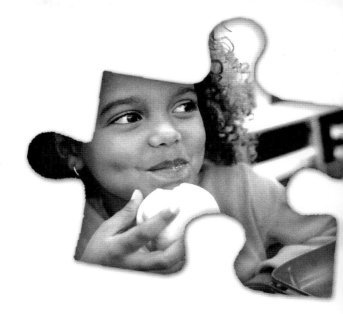

Summary

If local government officials were asked to describe their vision of what a healthy community looks like, they would probably cite many similar characteristics: effective and active schools; safe neighborhoods; clean parks and public spaces; and readily accessible services such as playgrounds, recreational facilities, libraries, and grocery stores. They might also paint a picture of healthy, happy children playing outside with their friends, walking to school, and eating healthy meals and snacks with their families and schoolmates.

This vision of healthy communities—places that promote the health and well-being of their residents—is a guidepost for childhood obesity prevention efforts. Taking actions that can make this vision a reality for all communities will help reverse and end this national epidemic. Childhood obesity has increased dramatically over the last three decades, and conditions in many communities continue to act as barriers to healthy eating and adequate physical activity. Childhood obesity is a serious health problem that has adverse and potentially long-lasting consequences for individuals, families, and communities. Perhaps most shocking, life expectancy for today's children may be shortened in the United States because of the impact of childhood obesity (Olshansky and Ludwig, 2005).

The good news is that actions can be taken to prevent childhood obesity. Many of these actions, both policy and programmatic, can and should be taken at the local level. Two previous Institute of Medicine (IOM) reports take a comprehensive look at childhood obesity, present conclusions about likely causes and solutions, and offer recommendations for next steps (IOM, 2005, 2007). Many of these recommendations touch on the vital role of government actions at all levels—federal, state, and local—in childhood obesity prevention. Local government leadership is critical to both reducing and preventing further increases in childhood obesity. The places in which people live, work, study, and play have a strong influence on their ability to consume healthy foods and beverages and engage in regular physical activity. Local governments make decisions every day that affect these environments. Thus, this report focuses on specific actions for local governments and is meant to be a tool for use by local government officials—mayors, managers, commissioners, council members, or administrators; elected, appointed, or hired; at the city, town, township, or county level—in planning, implementing, and refining childhood obesity efforts in their jurisdictions.

In 2008, the IOM Standing Committee on Childhood Obesity identified local government actions as key to front-line efforts addressing obesity prevention and requested a study to examine the evidence on such local government efforts, with a focus on identifying promising practices and developing a set of recommended actions. That committee was inspired by the recommendations in the previous IOM reports on childhood obesity and by the clear need for more detail at the local government level on which specific actions have the potential to make a difference. The IOM Committee on Childhood Obesity Prevention Actions for Local Governments was formed to address this task. The committee entered this project knowing that evidence on the best childhood obesity prevention practices is still accumulating and is limited in many important areas. However, the committee also knew that many local government officials want to act now on the best available information.

The committee reviewed the published literature, examined reports from organizations that work with local government, invited presentations from experts on the role of local government in obesity prevention, and explored a variety of toolkits that have been developed for communities. The committee worked to develop actionable recommendations for promoting healthy eating and physical activity and guided its decisions toward actions that are within the jurisdiction of local governments; are likely to affect children directly; are based on the experience of local governments or knowledgeable sources that work with local governments; and have the potential to make positive contributions to the achievement of healthy eating and/or optimum physical activity based on research evidence or, where such evidence is lacking or limited, a logical connection with the achievement of healthier eating and increased physical activity. The committee developed a set of criteria to consider in assessing the actions to recommend. Using the best evidence available, the committee took into account effectiveness and effect size;

outcomes, including those not directly related to obesity prevention; potential reach, impact, and cost; and feasibility (see Appendix C).

In this report, *healthy eating* refers to consuming the types and amounts of foods, nutrients, and calories recommended by the Dietary Guidelines for Americans (HHS and USDA, 2005). In the area of physical activity, current recommendations are for children to engage in such activity at least 60 minutes per day (HHS and USDA, 2008).

The committee targeted its recommendations to the food and physical activity environments outside the school walls and the school day. What takes place inside schools from the morning bell to the end of the last class and its impact on childhood obesity has been widely discussed (IOM, 2005, 2007; Story et al., 2006). By contrast, many other aspects of children's environments, from the accessibility and maintenance of neighborhood playgrounds to the food and beverage choices offered in after-school programs, have not been discussed and publicized to the same extent. Therefore, the report generally focuses on nonschool issues. This focus does not imply that schools are unimportant in the prevention of childhood obesity. In fact, the involvement of schools in obesity prevention is vital; obesity prevention initiatives undertaken outside of schools will be stronger and have a greater impact if they are coordinated with and complement those of schools.

In this report, the committee recommends nine healthy eating strategies and six physical activity strategies that local governments should consider. These strategies are organized under three healthy eating goals and three physical activity goals. For each strategy, the report recommends a set of actions that have the potential to make a difference. The report also highlights 12 actions that the committee believes have the greatest potential, based on an assessment of the available research evidence and a logical connection with the achievement of healthier eating and increased physical activity. These 12 actions are highlighted in the list of goals, strategies, and actions at the end of this summary.

Evidence points to multisectoral initiatives (involving government, schools, the private sector, nonprofit organizations, and families) as being most effective in promoting and sustaining a healthy environment for children and youth (Economos et al., 2007; Sacks et al., 2008; Samuels and Associates, 2009). In many communities, however, policy makers may want to begin their obesity prevention efforts with some individual actions that they believe would be a good starting point, in preparation for later work on broader efforts.

While overall strategies can be recommended in accordance with evidence-based research, this information must be balanced with the need for community participation in defining what is needed. The local context—including resources, demographics, culture, geographic location, and jurisdictional authority—will drive decisions on the policies and initiatives that can be implemented and sustained. While overall strategies can be recommended, and a range of potential actions to implement those strategies can be recommended, local officials and their community partners must use their own collective knowledge, judgment, and expertise to choose the best actions for their locality. Actions chosen must be a good fit for the community, and local government officials must be able to convince supporters and funders that these steps are important.

As local government officials work to understand the characteristics, needs, and assets of their communities, it will be critically important to involve concerned community members in examining, recommending, and building support for particular actions. These community members should include, among many others, parents, youth, and health providers. In addition, it will be important to partner with neighborhood-based grassroots nonprofit organizations, since they often have established networks for communication and outreach to residents. Active leadership is also key, and many mayors, city council representatives, and others have already taken the initiative to be prominently engaged in leading community efforts and involving community coalitions in promoting access to and availability of healthy choices and a healthy environment for their community.

Particular attention should be paid to conditions that result in unequal access to opportunities for healthy foods and beverages and physical activity. Factors such as poverty, poor housing, racial segregation, lack of access to quality education, and limited access to health care can influence access to healthy food and physical activity in negative ways. Understanding this interrelationship in the case of childhood obesity could lead local officials to note that many lower-income children in their jurisdiction do not engage in physical activity, and consequently to examine the equity of access to parks and recreational opportunities and safe neighborhoods and work to end these inequities. Local officials might observe inadequate consumption of fruits and vegetables among children in some parts of the community, and then consider and seek solutions to the unequal accessibility and affordability of healthy foods in these neighborhoods. Achieving health equity—"the fair distribution of health determinants, outcomes, and resources within and between segments of the population regardless of social standing" (CDC, 2007)—requires local governments to focus their obesity prevention efforts on historically disadvantaged communities with disproportionately high rates of obesity.

Finally, as obesity prevention actions are implemented, they will need to be evaluated. Local governments can contribute to the evidence base on what does and does not work by emphasizing and funding assessments of obesity prevention efforts. Partnerships with local universities can be particularly valuable in conducting these evaluations. Lessons learned through experimentation and formal evaluation can assist a community in making better decisions about future actions while helping other communities like them become more successful in preventing childhood obesity.

REFERENCES

CDC (Centers for Disease Control and Prevention). 2007 (unpublished). *Health Equity Working Group*. Atlanta, GA: CDC.

Economos, C. D., R. R. Hyatt, J. P. Goldberg, A. Must, E. N. Naumova, J. J. Collins, and M. E. Nelson. 2007. A community intervention reduces BMI z-score in children: Shape Up Somerville first year results. *Obesity* 15(5):1325–1336.

HHS and USDA (U.S. Department of Health and Human Services and U.S. Department of Agriculture). 2005. *Dietary Guidelines for Americans 2005*. http://www.healthierus. gov/dietaryguidelines (accessed February 25, 2009).

HHS and USDA. 2008. *Physical Activity Guidelines for Americans*. http://www.health.gov/ paguidelines/guidelines/default.aspx (accessed May 19, 2009).

IOM (Institute of Medicine). 2005. *Preventing Childhood Obesity: Health in the Balance*. Washington, DC: The National Academies Press.

IOM. 2007. *Progress in Preventing Childhood Obesity: How Do We Measure Up?* Washington, DC: The National Academies Press.

Olshansky, S. J., and D. S. Ludwig. 2005. Effect of obesity on life expectancy in the U.S. *Food Technology* 59(7):112.

Sacks, G., B. A. Swinburn, and M. A. Lawrence. 2008. A systematic policy approach to changing the food system and physical activity environments to prevent obesity. *Australia and New Zealand Health Policy* 5.

Samuels and Associates. 2009. *Healthy Eating, Active Communities (HEAC) Phase 1 Evaluation Findings, 2005–2008. Executive Summary*. http://samuelsandassociates.com/ samuels/index.php?option=com_content&view=article&id=27&Itemid=11 (accessed July 13, 2009).

Story, M., K. M. Kaphingst, and S. French. 2006. The role of schools in obesity prevention. *Future of Children* 16(1):109–142.

Actions for Healthy Eating

(**Bold** denotes most promising action steps)

GOAL 1: IMPROVE ACCESS TO AND CONSUMPTION OF HEALTHY, SAFE, AND AFFORDABLE FOODS

Strategy 1: Retail Outlets

Increase community access to healthy foods through supermarkets, grocery stores, and convenience/corner stores.

Action Steps

- **Create incentive programs to attract supermarkets and grocery stores to underserved neighborhoods (e.g., tax credits, grant and loan programs, small business/economic development programs, and other economic incentives).**
- Realign bus routes or provide other transportation, such as mobile community vans or shuttles to ensure that residents can access supermarkets or grocery stores easily and affordably through public transportation.
- Create incentive programs to enable current small food store owners in underserved areas to carry healthier, affordable food items (e.g., grants or loans to purchase refrigeration equipment to store fruits, vegetables, and fat-free/low-fat dairy; free publicity; a city awards program; or linkages to wholesale distributors).
- Use zoning regulations to enable healthy food providers to locate in underserved neighborhoods (e.g., "as of right" and "conditional use permits").
- Enhance accessibility to grocery stores through public safety efforts, such as better outdoor lighting and police patrolling.

Strategy 2: Restaurants

Improve the availability and identification of healthful foods in restaurants.

Action Steps

- **Require menu labeling in chain restaurants to provide consumers with calorie information on in-store menus and menu boards.**
- Encourage non-chain restaurants to provide consumers with calorie information on in-store menus and menu boards.
- Offer incentives (e.g., recognition or endorsement) for restaurants that promote healthier options (for example, by increasing the offerings of healthier foods, serving age-appropriate portion sizes, or making the default standard options healthy—i.e., apples or carrots instead of French fries, and non-fat milk instead of soda in "kids' meals").

Strategy 3: Community Food Access

Promote efforts to provide fruits and vegetables in a variety of settings, such as farmers' markets, farm stands, mobile markets, community gardens, and youth-focused gardens.

Action Steps

- Encourage farmers markets to accept Special Supplemental Nutrition Program for Women, Infants and Children (WIC) food package vouchers and WIC Farmers Market Nutrition Program coupons; and encourage and make it possible for farmers markets to accept Supplemental Nutrition Assistance Program (or SNAP, formerly the Food Stamp Program) and WIC Program Electronic Benefit Transfer (EBT) cards by allocating funding for equipment that uses electronic methods of payment.
- Improve funding for outreach, education, and transportation to encourage use of farmers' markets and farm stands by residents of lower-income neighborhoods, and by WIC and SNAP recipients.
- Introduce or modify land use policies/zoning regulations to promote, expand, and protect potential sites for community gardens and farmers' markets, such as vacant city-owned land or unused parking lots.
- Develop community-based group activities (e.g., community kitchens) that link procurement of affordable, healthy food with improving skills in purchasing and preparing food.

Strategy 4: Public Programs and Worksites

Ensure that publicly run entities such as after-school programs, child care facilities, recreation centers, and local government worksites implement policies and practices to promote healthy foods and beverages and reduce or eliminate the availability of calorie-dense, nutrient-poor foods.

Action Steps

- **Mandate and implement strong nutrition standards for foods and beverages available in government-run or regulated after-school programs, recreation centers, parks, and child care facilities (which includes limiting access to calorie-dense, nutrient-poor foods).**
- Ensure that local government agencies that operate cafeterias and vending options have strong nutrition standards in place wherever foods and beverages are sold or available.
- Provide incentives or subsidies to government-run or -regulated programs and localities that provide healthy foods at competitive prices and limit calorie-dense, nutrient-poor foods (e.g., after-school programs that provide fruits or vegetables every day, and eliminate calorie-dense, nutrient-poor foods in vending machines or as part of the program).

Strategy 5: Government Nutrition Programs

Increase participation in federal, state, and local government nutrition assistance programs (e.g., WIC, School Breakfast and Lunch Programs, the Child and Adult Care Food Program, the Afterschool Snacks Program, the Summer Food Service Program, SNAP).

Action Steps

- Put policies in place that require government-run and -regulated agencies responsible for administering nutrition assistance programs to collaborate across agencies and programs to increase enrollment and participation in these programs (i.e., WIC agencies should ensure that those who are eligible are also participating in SNAP, etc.).
- Ensure that child care and after-school program licensing agencies encourage utilization of the nutrition assistance programs and increase nutrition program enrollment (CACFP, Afterschool Snack Program, and the Summer Food Service Program).

Strategy 6: Breastfeeding

Encourage breastfeeding and promote breastfeeding-friendly communities.

Action Steps

- Adopt practices in city and county hospitals that are consistent with the Baby-Friendly Hospital Initiative USA (United Nations Children's Fund/World Health Organization). This initiative promotes, protects, and supports breastfeeding through 10 steps to successful breastfeeding for hospitals.
- Permit breastfeeding in public places and rescind any laws or regulations that discourage or do not allow breastfeeding in public places and encourage the creation of lactation rooms in public places.
- Develop incentive programs to encourage government agencies to ensure breastfeeding-friendly worksites, including providing lactation rooms.
- Allocate funding to WIC clinics to acquire breast pumps to loan to participants.

Strategy 7: Access to Drinking Water

Increase access to free, safe drinking water in public places to encourage consumption of water instead of sugar-sweetened beverages.

Action Steps

- Require that plain water be available in local government-operated and administered outdoor areas and other public places and facilities.
- **Adopt building codes to require access to, and maintenance of, fresh drinking water fountains (e.g., public restroom codes).**

GOAL 2: REDUCE ACCESS TO AND CONSUMPTION OF CALORIE-DENSE, NUTRIENT-POOR FOODS

Strategy 8: Policies and Ordinances

Implement fiscal policies and local ordinances that discourage the consumption of calorie-dense, nutrient-poor foods and beverages (e.g., taxes, incentives, land use and zoning regulations).

Action Steps

- **Implement a tax strategy to discourage consumption of foods and beverages that have minimal nutritional value, such as sugar-sweetened beverages.**
- Adopt land use and zoning policies that restrict fast food establishments near school grounds and public playgrounds.
- Implement local ordinances to restrict mobile vending of calorie-dense, nutrient-poor foods near schools and public playgrounds.
- Implement zoning designed to limit the density of fast food establishments in residential communities.
- Eliminate advertising and marketing of calorie-dense, nutrient-poor foods and beverages near school grounds and public places frequently visited by youths.
- Create incentive and recognition programs to encourage grocery stores and convenience stores to reduce point-of-sale marketing of calorie-dense, nutrient-poor foods (i.e., promote "candy-free" check out aisles and spaces).

GOAL 3: RAISE AWARENESS ABOUT THE IMPORTANCE OF HEALTHY EATING TO PREVENT CHILDHOOD OBESITY

Strategy 9: Media and Social Marketing

Promote media and social marketing campaigns on healthy eating and childhood obesity prevention.

Action Steps

- **Develop media campaigns, utilizing multiple channels (print, radio, Internet, television, social networking, and other promotional materials) to promote healthy eating (and active living) using consistent messages.**
- Design a media campaign that establishes community access to healthy foods as a health equity issue and reframes obesity as a consequence of environmental inequities and not just the result of poor personal choices.
- Develop counter-advertising media approaches against unhealthy products to reach youth as has been used in the tobacco and alcohol prevention fields.

Actions for Increasing Physical Activity

(**Bold** denotes most promising action steps)

GOAL 1: ENCOURAGE PHYSICAL ACTIVITY

Strategy 1: Built Environment

Encourage walking and bicycling for transportation and recreation through improvements in the built environment.

Action Steps

- Adopt a pedestrian and bicycle master plan to develop a long-term vision for walking and bicycling in the community and guide implementation.
- **Plan, build, and maintain a network of sidewalks and street crossings that creates a safe and comfortable walking environment and that connects to schools, parks, and other destinations.**
- Plan, build, and retrofit streets so as to reduce vehicle speeds, accommodate bicyclists, and improve the walking environment.
- Plan, build, and maintain a well-connected network of off-street trails and paths for pedestrians and bicyclists.
- Increase destinations within walking and bicycling distance.
- Collaborate with school districts and developers to build new schools in locations central to residential areas and away from heavily trafficked roads.

Strategy 2: Programs for Walking and Biking

Promote programs that support walking and bicycling for transportation and recreation.

Action Steps

- **Adopt community policing strategies that improve safety and security of streets, especially in higher crime neighborhoods.***
- **Collaborate with schools to develop and implement a Safe Routes to School program to increase the number of children safely walking and bicycling to schools.**
- Improve access to bicycles, helmets, and related equipment for lower-income families, for example, through subsidies or repair programs.
- Promote increased transit use through reduced fares for children, families, and students, and improved service to schools, parks, recreation centers, and other family destinations.
- Implement a traffic enforcement program to improve safety for pedestrians and bicyclists.

---

*Two action steps on community policing were combined for the most promising 12 action steps list.

Local Government Actions to Prevent Childhood Obesity

Strategy 3: Recreational Physical Activity

Promote other forms of recreational physical activity.

Action Steps

- **Build and maintain parks and playgrounds that are safe and attractive for playing, and in close proximity to residential areas.**
- **Adopt community policing strategies that improve safety and security for park use, especially in higher crime neighborhoods.***
- Improve access to public and private recreational facilities in communities with limited recreational options through reduced costs, increased operating hours, and development of culturally appropriate activities.
- Create after-school activity programs (e.g., dance classes, city-sponsored sports, supervised play, and other publicly or privately supported active recreation).
- **Collaborate with school districts and other organizations to establish joint use of facilities agreements allowing playing fields, playgrounds, and recreation centers to be used by community residents when schools are closed; if necessary, adopt regulatory and legislative policies to address liability issues that might block implementation.**
- Create and promote youth athletic leagues and increase access to fields, with special emphasis on income and gender equity.
- Build and provide incentives to build recreation centers in neighborhoods.

Strategy 4: Routine Physical Activity

Promote policies that build physical activity into daily routines.

Action Steps

- **Institute regulatory policies mandating minimum play space, physical equipment, and duration of play in preschool, after-school, and child care programs.**
- Develop worksite policies and practices that build physical activity into routines (for example, exercise breaks at a certain time of day and in meetings or walking meetings). Target worksites with high percentages of youth employees and government-run and -regulated worksites.
- Create incentives for remote parking and drop-off zones and/or disincentives for nearby parking and drop-off zones at schools, public facilities, shopping malls, and other destinations.
- Improve stairway access and appeal, especially in places frequented by children.

---

*Two action steps on community policing were combined for the most promising 12 action steps list.

GOAL 2: DECREASE SEDENTARY BEHAVIOR

Strategy 5: Screen Time

Promote policies that reduce sedentary screen time.

Action Steps

- Adopt regulatory policies limiting screen time in preschool and after-school programs.

GOAL 3: RAISE AWARENESS OF THE IMPORTANCE OF INCREASING PHYSICAL ACTIVITY

Strategy 6: Media and Social Marketing

Develop a social marketing campaign that emphasizes the multiple benefits for children and families of sustained physical activity.

Action Steps

- Develop media campaigns, utilizing multiple channels (print, radio, Internet, television, other promotional materials) to promote physical activity using consistent messages.
- Design a media campaign that establishes physical activity as a health equity issue and reframes obesity as a consequence of environmental inequities and not just the result of poor personal choices.
- Develop counter-advertising media approaches against sedentary activity to reach youth as has been done in the tobacco and alcohol prevention fields.

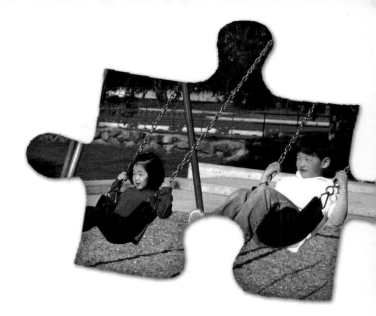

Introduction

The topic of this report was recommended by the Institute of Medicine's (IOM's) Standing Committee on Childhood Obesity Prevention. The report grew out of an experience of one of the committee members who was approached by a local city council member with this request: "I want to do something about the increasing problem of childhood obesity in our city. What are the top prevention strategies I should pursue?" Although a well-versed obesity researcher, this committee member was struck by the challenges involved in answering the council member's question. This report is designed to respond to those challenges and provide information to local government officials who are choosing childhood obesity prevention strategies for their communities.

To that end, the IOM convened a committee charged with examining the range of childhood obesity prevention efforts that have been considered or implemented by local governments, with a focus on identifying promising practices that could serve as the basis for a set of recommendations for dissemination to local government officials and entities. The audience for the report was to include mayors; county, city, or township commissioners or other officials; local health departments; local boards of health; city and transportation planners; and other relevant local commissions and public entities. The committee was asked to draw from and build on relevant IOM reports, as well as secondary sources and seminal primary sources. The committee was to note promising strategies for addressing disparities and disproportionately affected children and youth, identify other public health benefits of obesity prevention initiatives, and summarize successful strategies for sustained funding and financing of such initiatives. Thus the committee was charged with developing a succinct report that would summarize the range of local government efforts, identify and describe the rationale for selected promising practices, discuss other relevant public health benefits of these practices, and present a set of recommendations for actions for local governments to consider in addressing childhood obesity. (See Appendix E for the official Statement of Task for the committee.)

PURPOSE OF THE REPORT

Trends in Childhood Obesity

The city council member who approached the committee member with his urgent request for advice was right to be concerned. The health and well-being of children in the United States are threatened by the ever-increasing number and percentage who are overweight and obese—now at one in four children. Childhood and adolescent obesity has increased dramatically in just three decades. Among children aged 2–5, the prevalence of obesity has increased from 5 percent to 12.4 percent; among children aged 6–11, it has increased from 6.5 percent to 17 percent; and among adolescents (aged 12–19), it has more than tripled, from 5 percent to 17.6 percent (CDC, NHANES) (Figure 1-1). Overall, more than 16.3 percent of children and adolescents aged 2–19 are obese (Ogden et al., 2008). And while children in all race/ethnicity and socioeconomic groups are increasingly obese, those in some groups (the poor, African Americans, Latinos, American Indians, and Pacific Islanders) are disproportionately more overweight and obese.

Obesity is so prevalent that it may reduce the life expectancy of today's generation of children and diminish the overall quality of their lives (Olshansky and Ludwig, 2005). This is because obese children and adolescents are more likely to have hypertension, high cholesterol, and type 2 diabetes when they are young (Daniels, 2009; Gunturu and Ten, 2007), and they also are more likely to be obese when they are adults (Freedman et al., 2009).

A Tool for Local Governments

Much has been written about the epidemic of childhood obesity and strategies for reversing current trends. Two previous IOM reports, *Preventing Childhood Obesity: Health in the Balance* and *Progress in Preventing Childhood Obesity: How Do We Measure Up?*, consider the issue of childhood obesity and present recommendations for consideration both generally and by specific groups or audiences (IOM, 2005,

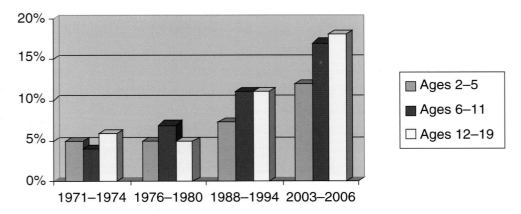

FIGURE 1-1 Prevalence of obesity among children, 1971–2006.
SOURCE: CDC, NHANES.

2007). Those recommendations call for governmental leadership, at all levels, on better measurement of childhood obesity; consideration of the unique characteristics and contexts of people in communities when obesity prevention initiatives are being developed; evaluation of programs to see what works; and dissemination of information about what does and does not work. This report is meant to serve as a tool for local government officials, mayors, managers, commissioners, council members, or administrators; elected, appointed, or hired; at the city, town, township, or county level—and those who work in partnership with them to help in tackling the prevention of childhood obesity in their jurisdictions.

Tip O'Neill, former Speaker of the U.S. House of Representatives, is credited with having said that "all politics is local." All health is local as well. Health is, first of all, a personal matter. It is very "local" and extends outward from the individual to include the family, close relationships, and the community. Second, although health is strongly influenced by state, regional, national, and international trends and actions, many strategies for addressing childhood obesity must be carried out at the local level to make a difference.

An old adage says that a healthy child is a happy child. Likewise, a fit student is a better-performing student (Chomitz et al., 2009; Mahar et al., 2006). Whether by casual observation or more scientific study, it is clear that the overall well-being of a child affects his or her behavior and academic performance. While much has been done by the nation and at the community level to improve the health prospects of children through public health and medical interventions such as prenatal care, immunizations, and provision of antibiotics, the growing prevalence of childhood overweight and obesity is threatening the gains made in child health over the past decades.

The causes of childhood obesity are complex. Although the simple explanation is that too many calories are ingested (through consumption of food and beverages) and too few calories are expended (through physical activity), the physiological solution (a balance of the amount of calories consumed and used) is more than a matter of individual willpower or personal responsibility. Living in an environment that lacks healthy food choices and encourages unhealthy ones is a challenge to overcome. An environment that offers no place to play and nowhere safe to walk is likely to discourage optimum physical activity. Even the most motivated adult or parent, or the best-trained child, can find it difficult to act in healthy ways if the surrounding environment does not support or even allow such activity. Thus the real solutions to obesity must take into consideration the environments in which children live, learn, and play. The characteristics of these environments, such as the availability of healthy foods and beverages, the safety of streets, and the accessibility of recreation opportunities, can have a strong impact on whether children become obese. By helping to change these environments in positive ways, local governments can enable families and children to act to maintain and improve their health and prevent the development of obesity.

Childhood obesity prevention in the school setting, during the school day, has received a great deal of attention in particular. Students spend much of their time at school, which thus provides many opportunities for improving food and beverage consumption and levels of physical activity. Many other crucial aspects of children's environments have not been talked about and publicized to the same extent. Thus, the focus of this report is on actions that local governments can take outside of the school setting, and outside of school hours, to prevent childhood obesity. Local governments can do a great deal to bring positive changes to these other environments. These changes can influence how healthy the food and beverages consumed outside of school are (e.g., in after-school programs) and the extent to which children engage in physical activity, which can depend on the accessibility and maintenance of neighborhood playgrounds. By focusing on such broader environmental factors as well as on what happens during the school day, local governments are likely to increase their chances of success in preventing childhood obesity. This focus does not imply that schools are unimportant in the prevention of childhood obesity. In fact, the involvement of schools in obesity prevention is vital: Obesity prevention initiatives undertaken outside of schools will be stronger and have a greater impact if they are coordinated with and complement those within schools.

Evidence points to multisectoral initiatives as being effective in achieving and sustaining prevention of childhood obesity (Economos et al., 2007; Sacks et al., 2008; Samuels and Associates, 2009). However, some local government officials may start by implementing one or several programs and/or policies that they believe will help prevent obesity, are easily doable, and will receive community support. At a future date, communities may develop a more comprehensive childhood obesity prevention plan that involves every department and program within local government, businesses, community organizations, schools, families, and individuals. A multisectoral plan can include clear roles, responsibilities, and policies that make the healthy choices the easy choices by giving communities, schools, businesses, and families the tools they need to make it easier to follow national recommendations for healthy eating and physical activity.

APPROACH TO IDENTIFYING PROMISING ACTIONS

Guiding Principles

The committee developed a set of principles to guide its deliberations on promising actions. These principles are summarized in Box 1-1 and detailed below.

1. Childhood obesity prevention is crucial to the future health of the nation.

Childhood obesity poses a serious threat to health in the United States. Obesity is associated with increased disability, disease, and death and has substantial health, economic, and social costs (IOM, 2007). Therefore, addressing childhood obesity could be one of the most powerful means to improve the health of the nation. A review of health trends suggests that illness, disability, early death, and medical costs will increase if nothing is done now to prevent and reverse childhood obesity (HHS, 2001). In addition, the present realities for obese children and their families are difficult because of the early onset of chronic diseases such as diabetes and the stigma associated with being a heavy child. At the same time, many children and youth have limited access to healthy foods and beverages and to places and opportunities to be physically active, along with too much access to energy-dense, low-nutrition foods and sedentary activities. Because of these concerns, local governments and policy makers bear a responsibility to children and families in their jurisdictions to enact policies that promote healthy eating and safe physical activity while discouraging unhealthy behaviors, much as they do with tobacco use and consumption of alcoholic beverages.

2. The creation of environments that support health is essential to preventing childhood obesity.

Parents and caregivers play a fundamental role in teaching children about healthy choices and behaviors, in modeling those behaviors, and in making decisions for children. However, the positive efforts of adults can be undermined by the environments in which children spend the rest of their time if these environments do not support engaging in healthy behaviors (IOM, 2005, 2007). For parents to succeed in raising healthy children and enable healthy choices to be made more easily, the surrounding environments must make such choices possible and easy.

3. Local government efforts are critical in childhood obesity prevention.

Local governments have a substantial influence in shaping policies and practices that influence the environments where children live, play, and learn and thereby affect their health. Federal and state policies addressing childhood obesity will, in most instances, be implemented at the local level; in addition, local policy makers and leaders will respond to the needs and priorities of their communities. Each community is different in its geography; demographics; and assets, such as fiscal capacity, nonprofit agency support, existence of willing partners in academia, and interest by the business community. A primary responsibility of local governments is to address health, safety, and education through policy and environmental changes. Historically, local governments have promoted children's health through public health initiatives, from ensuring that children are immunized to mandating bicycle helmets. In the same way, local governments can promote children's health by taking action to prevent childhood obesity.

4. Eliminating health disparities and achieving health equity should be priorities in any childhood obesity prevention effort.

Many local policies and environments fail to ensure equal access to places, resources, services, or support for all populations. The result is disparities in the prevalence of childhood obesity and in related health, social, and behavioral concerns. Given that the rates of childhood obesity are highest among lower-income and some racial/ethnic populations, local governments should consider giving priority to policy and environment strategies that minimize health inequities.

5. Collaboration and strong partnerships are key to childhood obesity prevention efforts at the local level.

To address childhood obesity effectively, strong partnerships and collaborations among a diverse set of community members are needed, both within and outside of government. Local governments are in a unique position to catalyze, support, or lead collaborations in the community and engage multiple constituents. Examples include health department staff working collaboratively with elected officials, city planners, school boards, traffic engineers, smart-growth representatives, community health and land use advocates, academia, local businesses, and other community organizations.

6. Evaluation at the local level is vital to understanding what works.

The evidence for local government policies that prevent childhood obesity is still accumulating. At the same time, communities need to identify and implement initiatives that can have a positive effect on nutrition and physical activity, and not wait to act until all the evidence is collected and published. There is a great need for communities to pursue evaluation activities in order to improve and expand the evidence base.

7. *It is important to consider potential negative and positive consequences of local government policies.*

Policy and environmental strategies that are not specifically focused on childhood obesity may nonetheless influence behaviors related to childhood obesity. Therefore, attention needs to be paid to potential impacts on healthy eating and physical activity before deciding whether to implement any policy or environmental strategy or to change past policies. Likewise, obesity prevention policies may have other effects unrelated to obesity. For example, a cooking program or recreation program after school may be initiated to prevent obesity, but these same programs also may help prevent crime during after-school hours by keeping youth engaged and safe. These additional positive effects may bring broader support to the obesity prevention efforts of local government, such as enthusiastic support for after-school programs among local police departments working to prevent crime among youth.

8. *Long-term benefits of childhood obesity prevention actions should be recognized and valued.*

Implementing policy and environmental strategies with long-term benefits, such as zoning restrictions, pedestrian master plans, or tax incentives to attract grocery stores to lower-income neighborhoods, can be complex or require considerable investments. These strategies have the potential to impact population changes in eating and activity behaviors, but implementation and positive outcomes may take time.

How the Action Steps Were Selected

Local governments are looking for the most effective actions they can take to prevent childhood obesity in their communities. As noted above, while the evidence base for local government actions is growing, limitations of current research should not discourage action. As highlighted in a 2005 IOM report, childhood obesity prevention actions "should be based on the best available evidence—as opposed to waiting for the best possible evidence" (IOM, 2005, p. 3). Local government officials need the benefit of the best available information to make the wisest possible decisions on action.

To assist in determining the most promising actions for local governments to take to prevent childhood obesity, the committee reviewed numerous articles from peer-reviewed journals, as well as reports from organizations that work with local governments on childhood obesity prevention. A broad spectrum of potential actions was identified, and the research results were compiled. In addition, several sets of criteria and tools developed by others to evaluate local childhood obesity prevention actions were examined. Informed by these efforts, the committee developed criteria for consideration as it made determinations about the most promising actions. See Appendixes B and C and the references in Chapters 4 and 5 for more details on the methodology used and the evidence identified.

The committee selected actions to recommend that local governments generally have the authority to carry out. In addition, actions had to have a direct impact on childhood obesity. This is somewhat of a gray area, since children live in families and are directly influenced by adults, but the committee attempted to focus its recommendations on those that can have the most direct effects on children. Also, as mentioned earlier, the committee focused on changes outside of the school setting and school day. (For example, the committee recommends Safe Routes to School programs, but did not examine physical education requirements during the school day.) In addition, actions had to have been implemented by local governments or recommended by knowledgeable sources as actions for local governments. Finally, the recommended actions had to be likely to make positive contributions to the achievement of healthy eating and/or optimal physical activity based on research evidence or, where that was lacking or limited, have a logical connection with the achievement of healthier eating or increased physical activity.

Once the committee determined the recommended action steps based on the methodology described above, it considered whether to rank the action steps according to the strength of research evidence (i.e., types and amount of evidence, and effect sizes) and/or by some other criterion. As mentioned earlier in this report, the evidence about childhood obesity prevention is still accumulating, and is limited in a number of areas. Yet, as this report highlights, there are many promising actions that can be pursued by local governments. Actions that are promising should not be automatically dismissed because of limited research. Moreover, priorities for action on childhood obesity prevention may vary from community to community depending on the local context. Local governments will take many things into account as they decide which action steps to take. Even the cost of an action will vary depending on community assets, and sometimes relative costs will be of secondary importance to the potential reach of an action step or the community support for it. Therefore, the committee did not rank its recommended action steps by the strength of evidence, effect sizes, or other criteria.

However, the report does include Appendix D, which focuses on the nature of the evidence supporting the action steps under each of the strategies. This appendix is included for those readers who are particularly interested in the evidence behind the action steps.

Finally, the committee did decide to highlight 12 of the action steps for special consideration. Although all of the recommended actions have a potential to make a difference, these 12 are the actions that were rated as most promising based on the criteria described in this chapter and in Appendix C.

First Steps

Before any efforts are undertaken to develop new programs or policies on obesity prevention, a survey should be conducted to understand local obesity prevention efforts already under way. It is important to talk with people in the community, organizations, or current government programs that have efforts in progress. These partners can help local officials identify what is needed for obesity prevention and how local government can help build on existing efforts. A partnership between local officials and those involved in obesity prevention efforts is critical for sustainability.

After surveying existing efforts, local governments will need to decide how to take the first step. While many actions are recommended in this report, there are also many simple first steps that local government officials can take to get started on preventing childhood obesity in their communities. The committee compiled a list of 10 simple first steps, each of which could serve as a starting point for local officials (Box 1-2).

ORGANIZATION OF THE REPORT

This report is organized to support decision making by local government officials, staff, and collaborators on childhood obesity prevention actions. Recognizing that each community is unique, the second chapter reviews local issues that should be considered in making decisions about childhood obesity prevention strategies. The third chapter addresses the importance of recognizing, understanding, and resolving disparities in the prevalence of obesity and its causes. Chapters 4 and 5 are the core of the report: a discussion and listing of promising childhood obesity prevention strategies and actions to promote healthy eating and increased physical activity. Those actions that the committee deems most promising are highlighted.

Box 1-2
10 Simple First Steps

1. Ask your planning director to take a walk with you on the best and the least pedestrian-friendly streets in your jurisdiction.
2. Have lunch with your health director to discuss childhood obesity prevention.
3. Post a blog entry asking the community for ideas for reducing childhood obesity.
4. Propose that the next appointment to your planning board be selected from a pool of applicants that will provide a health perspective.
5. Contact your state and national associations for an update on the latest work they are doing on childhood obesity.
6. Look at the child care licensing regulations in your community and see whether nutrition and physical activity are adequately addressed.
7. Check with your state department of transportation on the requirements, process, and deadlines for applying for funding from the federal Safe Routes to School program.
8. Ask the health department to analyze numbers from any available surveillance data aggregated, for example, by city council or supervisorial district. The results might help local elected and appointed officials understand existing health disparities in their community.
9. Ask your police chief what could be done to enforce existing pedestrian safety laws or what new laws might be needed.
10. Review bus routes and schedules to see whether changing them could make parks, recreation centers, and supermarkets more accessible.

REFERENCES

CDC (Centers for Disease Control and Prevention). *National Health and Nutrition Examination Survey (NHANES)*. http://www.cdc.gov/nchs/about/major/nhanes/datalink.htm (accessed May 20, 2009).

Chomitz, V. R., M. M. Slining, R. J. McGowan, S. E. Mitchell, G. F. Dawson, and K. A. Hacker. 2009. Is there a relationship between physical fitness and academic achievement? Positive results from public school children in the northeastern United States. *Journal of School Health* 79(1):30–37.

Daniels, S. R. 2009. Complications of obesity in children and adolescents. *International Journal of Obesity* 33(Suppl. 1):S60–S65.

Economos, C. D., R. R. Hyatt, J. P. Goldberg, A. Must, E. N. Naumova, J. J. Collins, and M. E. Nelson. 2007. A community intervention reduces BMI z-score in children: Shape Up Somerville first year results. *Obesity* 15(5):1325–1336.

Freedman, D. S., W. H. Dietz, S. R. Srinivasan, and G. S. Berenson. 2009. Risk factors and adult body mass index among overweight children: The Bogalusa heart study. *Pediatrics* 123(3):750–757.

Gunturu, S. D., and S. Ten. 2007. Complications of obesity in childhood. *Pediatric Annals* 36(2):96–101.

HHS (U.S. Department of Health and Human Services). 2001. *The Surgeon General's Call to Action to Prevent and Decrease Overweight and Obesity.* http://www.surgeongeneral. gov/topics/obesity/calltoaction/CalltoAction.pdf (accessed May 12, 2009).

IOM (Institute of Medicine). 2005. *Preventing Childhood Obesity: Health in the Balance.* Washington, DC: The National Academies Press.

IOM. 2007. *Progress in Preventing Childhood Obesity: How Do We Measure Up?* Washington, DC: The National Academies Press.

Mahar, M. T., S. K. Murphy, D. A. Rowe, J. Golden, A. T. Shields, and T. D. Raedeke. 2006. Effects of a classroom-based program on physical activity and on-task behavior. *Medicine and Science in Sports and Exercise* 38(12):2086–2094.

Ogden, C. L., M. D. Carroll, and K. M. Flegal. 2008. High body mass index for age among U.S. children and adolescents, 2003–2006. *Journal of the American Medical Association* 299(20):2401–2405.

Olshansky, S. J., and D. S. Ludwig. 2005. Effect of obesity on life expectancy in the U.S. *Food Technology* 59(7):112.

Sacks, G., B. A. Swinburn, and M. A. Lawrence. 2008. A systematic policy approach to changing the food system and physical activity environments to prevent obesity. *Australia and New Zealand Health Policy* 5.

Samuels and Associates. 2009. *Healthy Eating, Active Communities (HEAC) Phase 1 Evaluation Findings, 2005–2008. Executive Summary.* http://samuelsandassociates.com/ samuels/index.php?option=com_content&view=article&id=27&Itemid=11 (accessed July 13, 2009).

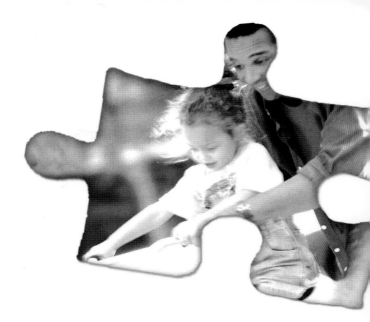

2

Acting Locally

Whether rural, suburban, or urban, most communities in the United States are affected by rising rates of childhood obesity. Healthy eating and physical activity are strongly associated with obesity prevention and are essential to good health. The food and physical activity choices made every day affect short- and long-term health and are directly related to weight outcomes. Eating right and being physically active may reduce the risk for heart disease, high blood pressure, diabetes, osteoporosis, certain cancers, and being overweight or obese (HHS and USDA, 2005). These diseases and conditions impact individuals and their quality of life and are associated with increasing health care costs that place a burden on government and businesses. Childhood provides the opportunity to establish a solid foundation that can lead to healthy lifelong eating patterns (IOM, 2005). Prevention of childhood obesity is essential to the promotion of a healthier and more productive society (IOM, 2005). In addition, many diet-related chronic diseases have their origins during childhood and adolescence.

Local governments make many of the decisions that affect access to healthy food and opportunities for physical activity and therefore play an important role in preventing childhood obesity. Because many children in cities and towns nationwide are facing the health and emotional consequences of childhood obesity, it is incumbent upon local governments to strengthen the role they play in providing their children and youth with access to and availability of healthy choices.

Local government agencies have traditionally been the primary overseers and implementers of public health programs and policies. The functions of local governments include leadership, provision of program resources, funding, evaluation, monitoring and research, and dissemination and use of evidence from evaluations (IOM, 2007). Local governments across the nation comprise a variety of departments, including public health, public works, transportation, parks and recreation, public safety, planning, economic development, housing, and tourism. These departments' policies and programs can affect childhood obesity directly and indirectly. For example, reducing vehicle traffic in a city for the purpose of reducing air pollution may also make it easier for people to walk to their destinations. Likewise, as noted in Chapter 1, policies and programs developed to prevent childhood obesity can meet other local government goals as well. For example, after-school recreation programs implemented to increase physical activity with obesity prevention in mind can help meet crime prevention goals by reducing opportunities for youth to be victims or perpetrators of crime. Since in some cases it is a great deal easier for a local government official to advocate for youth-related crime reduction measures than for childhood obesity prevention interventions, taking advantage of these multiple positive outcomes can be useful. Box 2-1 describes one city's sustainability plan that, although not focused explicitly on childhood obesity, contains many childhood obesity prevention strategies.

HOW LOCAL GOVERNMENTS CAN HELP

Provide Leadership

Local government leadership is critical to both reducing and preventing further increases in childhood obesity. Leadership requires galvanizing of political commitment, policy development, prioritized funding, and coordination of programs (Baker and Porter, 2005). Officials at the local level can work to adopt policies and pass ordinances that enable communities to have accessible and affordable options for healthy food and physical activity. Throughout the United States, mayors, city council members, and other local officials have initiated and led citywide campaigns and followed through on commitments to lead community walks and other fitness activities, in addition to providing leadership through innovative policy and program changes. Box 2-2 describes the example of a mayor who spearheaded a comprehensive health campaign in his small, rural town. Support for community coalitions focused on improving wellness is an additional key leadership contribution.

The City of Baltimore was named among the top ten most sustainable U.S. cities in SustainLane's 2008 U.S. City Rankings. Among the factors making Baltimore a national leader was the creation of the Baltimore Office of Sustainability and Commission on Sustainability. Baltimore Councilman Jim Kraft sponsored legislation to create both the office and the commission. The 21-member commission represents community organizations, local nonprofits, labor, private industry, local institutions, and city government. It was charged with developing and implementing a comprehensive Sustainability Plan to help turn Baltimore into a cleaner, greener, healthier, and safer city. The plan is a roadmap for future legislation, educational programming, and public and private initiatives involving sustainability.

The commission created working groups, community conversations, a youth strategy, and a sustainability forum to gather input from all sections and perspectives within Baltimore. Ultimately, more than 1,000 citizens were engaged over an eight-month period. The commission gathered and analyzed ideas, studied best practices, and developed goals for a more sustainable city. The resulting Sustainability Plan lays out 29 priority goals within seven chapters: Cleanliness, Pollution Prevention, Resource Conservation, Greening, Transportation, Education and Awareness, and Green Economy. Each of the 29 goals is accompanied by a set of recommended strategies.

The plan lays out a broad agenda that, in addition to recommending strategies for reducing pollution and conserving energy, offers recommendations for creating a healthier community. Many of these strategies relate to food access, transportation, and the built environment and so may help reduce and prevent obesity. Implementation of the plan not only will make Baltimore a cleaner, greener, healthier, and safer city, but also has the potential to reduce and prevent childhood obesity.

SOURCE: Baltimore Sustainability Plan, http://www.baltimorecity.gov/government/planning/sustainability.

Implement Policies, Ordinances, and Programs

Local governments are in a unique position to improve the health of their communities by advancing local policies that have an impact on the availability of healthy foods and places for physical activity and that also limit less healthy options. Local governments have jurisdiction over land use, food marketing, community planning, and transportation. Today, communities with the highest rates of obesity often are places where residents have the fewest convenient opportunities to purchase

Box 2-2
Comprehensive Obesity Prevention Efforts in a Rural Setting

Shelby is a rural town in eastern Montana with a population of approximately 3,000. Mayor Larry Bonderud has held his position for 18 years. After several years of attending conferences and reading about the environment and its effects on public health, Mayor Bonderud was inspired to make some significant city-wide changes. Like most rural towns, Shelby does not have a large public health budget. However, with the leadership of the mayor, the community has been able to initiate and implement a number of obesity prevention strategies:

- After surveying residents in the city newsletter, the mayor concluded that a fitness center was the first logical step for obesity prevention in Shelby. In partnership with a local hospital, he spearheaded an effort to install a fitness center in the local civic center and to hire a trainer. Memberships help sustain the center. The mayor and his community partners convinced major local employers to subsidize fitness center memberships for employees.

- The mayor and his committee of stakeholders planned a 6-mile paved walking trail that links the business district, residential neighborhoods, the Civic Center, the hospital, and schools to public lands. The trail was financed by the City of Shelby; the Community Transportation Enhancement Program; the Montana Fish, Wildlife and Parks Urban Recreational Trails Program; the Shelby Theme Committee; and in-kind contributions of labor and materials. Social marketing campaigns are being used to promote the trail.

- In partnership with others, the local health department developed a low-cost surveillance system to collect baseline data on breastfeeding rates in Shelby because of the strong association between breastfeeding and prevention of obesity later in life. The county public health nurse calls each new mother to see whether she needs information or resources. The nurse also asks if the mother is still breastfeeding, if she is feeding her child other foods, and if there are any factors that make it difficult to continue breastfeeding. The nurse repeats her calls quarterly. The county uses this information to help health care providers learn what interventions might increase breastfeeding initiation and duration.

- After surveying all Shelby households, Mayor Bonderud found that residents were overwhelmingly in favor of improving access to healthy foods in restaurants. He is working with Shelby restaurant managers and major food distributors to place healthier items on the menu. Once such items are in place, he hopes to conduct a promotional campaign aimed at encouraging residents to support those restaurants offering healthy food and to order the healthier items off the menu.

SOURCE: Baehr, 2008.

nutritious, affordable food and more opportunities to purchase less healthy choices (Flournoy and Treuhaft, 2005). As described in Chapter 4, relevant policy measures such as those focused on zoning of farmers' markets, location of supermarkets, limitations on advertising of unhealthy products, and requirements for menu labeling in restaurants all have the potential to affect consumption of fruits and vegetables and/or weight. Box 2-3 details how New York City enacted its menu labeling legislation, becoming the first city in the United States to mandate such labeling.

Similarly, Chapter 5 describes actions that local governments can take to increase physical activity through policy measures that affect the design of communities, access to parks and recreation facilities, and availability of sidewalks with safe pedestrian crossings. These actions affect the built environment, defined as all of the man-made elements of the physical environment, including buildings, infrastructure, and other physical elements created or modified by people, and the functional use, arrangement, and aesthetic qualities of these elements. The built environment can influence decisions on whether to be physically active. Evidence shows that people in activity-friendly environments are more likely to be physically active and have a lower risk of obesity (Frank et al., 2004). For example, children with sidewalks in their neighborhood and playgrounds in close proximity have more opportunities to be physically active. Local governments can influence community development and planning; zoning; and availability of, access to, and maintenance of parks and recreation facilities. In addition, reviewing transportation policies in a community can lead to improved access to opportunities for physical activity. Box 2-4 highlights the opportunities local governments have to provide support and resources to local organizations working to create healthy environments.

DIFFERENT COMMUNITIES, DIFFERENT NEEDS

As discussed in Chapter 1, each town, city, township, or community is unique, and only local government leaders can identify the policies and programs that accord with the resources and interests of their jurisdiction. Differences in geography, population, resources, and size present both challenges and opportunities for childhood obesity prevention efforts. Furthermore, local governance structures vary, differing in the extent of the local government's jurisdictional authority over schools, zoning, transportation policies, and many other issues. Sources of budget revenue and budget priorities and commitments also differ.

Rural, suburban, and urban communities all have different needs with respect to childhood obesity prevention. According to the U.S. Census,

Box 2-3
Menu Labeling Legislation

New York City has a population of more than 8 million, with millions of meals served in restaurants every day. In 2006, the New York City Board of Health unanimously voted to require chain restaurants to place calorie information on menus as a way to inform consumers about the health content of the food choices on the menu. New York City was the first city in the United States to require such action by restaurants. Menu labeling initiatives are being introduced across the country, but thus far, only New York City, Philadelphia, Seattle, Multnomah County in Oregon, and the states of California and Massachusetts have passed such legislation, and only New York City and Seattle have seen menu labeling go into effect. By April 2008, all chain restaurants in New York City with more than 15 outlets were required to include calorie information on menus and menu boards.

Since the 1960s, expenditure on foods eaten away from home has steadily increased (ERS, 2008). Eating out is associated with higher calorie intake and obesity (Duffey, 2007). Children consume almost twice as many calories when they eat restaurant meals compared with meals at home (770 vs. 420 calories) (Thompson et al., 2004). Many health professionals believe that menu labeling is a way for our "eating out" society to gain insight into restaurant food choices, just as nutrition labeling did for packaged foods. Studies have shown that most people cannot successfully estimate the calorie content of menu items, even when it comes to "healthy-sounding" items such as salads (Burton et al., 2006). Proponents believe that a consumer will choose healthier food if given nutrition information at the point of purchase. Some restaurants may even change the size or ingredients of menu items if required to display nutrition information.

Research is limited, but thus far supports this viewpoint. In a 2007 New York City survey, more than one-third of patrons at a popular fast-food restaurant that posts calorie information reported that this information affected their purchase. Patrons who saw the calorie information posted at the restaurant purchased, on average, food with 99 fewer calories compared with patrons who did not see that information posted (Basset et al., 2008). As more local health departments follow New York City's lead, there will be additional research on this possible obesity prevention strategy.

SOURCE: New York City Department of Health and Mental Hygiene, www.nyc.gov/html/doh.

Box 2-4
Encouraging Local Organizations to Be Fit

Austin, the capital of Texas, is a midsized city with a culturally diverse population of about 718,000. Austin is known for being socially progressive and health conscious, with its popular hike-and-bike trail, many farmers' markets, and the country's first Whole Foods supermarket. So Mayor Will Wynn was surprised to see Austin's poor ranking in a *Men's Fitness* magazine list of fittest cities a few years ago. He was inspired to form the Mayor's Fitness Council in October 2004 to help Austin become the fittest city in the country by 2010.

The council works toward increasing physical activity and improving nutrition throughout Austin. It consists of three committees that meet frequently to develop and implement programs. One such program is the Partner Certification Program, which encourages local organizations to help their employees or members become more fit. Certified Partners can include virtually any organization. Membership includes resident advocates from the public and private sectors, neighborhoods, schools, businesses, health care entities, and the faith-based community. Organizations can be certified by increasing:

- Access to smoke-free areas, fruits and vegetables, and opportunities for physical activity;
- Social support in the form of people participating together and encouraging each other in healthy behaviors;
- Incentives and rewards for people who engage in healthy behaviors;
- Decision prompts such as "Take the Stairs" signs near the elevators;
- Awareness through classes, e-mails, posters, etc.; and
- System changes such as cafeteria menu improvements.

The council developed the Austin Fitness Index, a survey tool that helps organizations monitor their employees' or members' health and track their improvements over time. The city assists companies that apply for the program in instituting programs and policy changes to help their employees become more fit. The city hopes that the benefits of increased employee health, such as better attitudes, productivity, and individual and organizational performance, will inspire many local organizations to become Certified Partners.

SOURCE: The Austin Fitness Index, http://www.ci.austin.tx.us/afi/default.htm.

approximately 55 million people (an estimated 20 percent of the U.S. population) live in rural communities spread across 85 percent of the United States. Children living in rural areas are recognized as being at high risk for childhood obesity (Dillon and Rowland, 2008); currently, 16.5 percent of rural children and 20.4 percent of rural adults are obese (Patterson et al., 2004). Challenges faced by some rural community residents include relative poverty; the need to travel long distances, requiring increased automobile use; fewer walking or biking routes; a lack of public transportation; and a lack of supermarkets.

Suburban communities are the fastest-growing areas in the United States. These communities have higher-density populations than rural communities, but may not always have convenient access to healthy food and opportunities for physical activity. Research has shown that several features of the suburban built environment, such as poor street connectivity and lack of sidewalks, are associated with decreased physical activity (Lopez and Hynes, 2006). However, new development offers the opportunity to plan healthier communities. The design of many new planned suburban communities includes "smart-growth" features such as sidewalks, parks, playgrounds, grocery stores and shops within walking distance, trails and bike paths, and easy access to public transportation.

Urban communities often have dense neighborhoods with excellent street connectivity, and streets almost always have sidewalks. Yet these communities also have poor economic conditions, unsafe streets, lack of access to nutritious food or grocery stores, and a high density of fast-food restaurants.

As each town or city government examines what it can do to promote health and wellness opportunities for its residents, it is important for local officials to consider the context and identify those strategies and actions most suited to their jurisdiction. Chapters 4 and 5 provide a broad array of actions from which local officials can choose to help initiate childhood obesity prevention efforts in their community. While a comprehensive approach is ideal, implementing even one or two actions could make an evident difference in the health of the community.

STEPS IN PLANNING LOCAL CHILDHOOD OBESITY PREVENTION EFFORTS

Local governments should consider the following steps as they plan childhood obesity prevention efforts:

1. Conduct a community assessment
2. Involve constituents
3. Identify top policy priorities best suited to local conditions

4.   Identify funding sources

5.   Think about program sustainability

6.   Evaluate programs and policies

1. Conduct a Community Assessment

Local government officials should consider initiating their efforts by conducting a community assessment of access to healthy food and opportunities for physical activity to determine where the community stands with respect to providing an optimal environment to support the healthy weight of children. Examples of community characteristics to include in this assessment are

- Location of grocery stores and supermarkets
- Location of fast-food restaurants
- Location of corner stores
- Location of vending machines
- Location of farmers' markets
- Location of food carts
- Location of water fountains in public facilities
- Extent of advertising of unhealthy food
- Statistics on and perceptions of safety
- Ease and safety of walking to school
- Location of walking and biking trails
- Condition and connectivity of sidewalks
- Condition and accessibility of youth activities and sports
- Location and availability of public transportation to grocery stores and recreational facilities
- Participation rates in federal nutrition assistance programs
- Location of community gardens

Using this and other relevant information, local governments can identify what features that promote healthy weight already exist in their community and what is still needed. Policies and programs can then be created to meet those needs.

In addition, it is important to identify resources and databases already in existence that can be used to learn more about the community. For example, information related to the health of the community can be drawn from a number of local government entities, including the zoning and planning department, the department of health, the tax assessor, schools and the transportation department, the county extension office, and mental health services. In addition, an academic

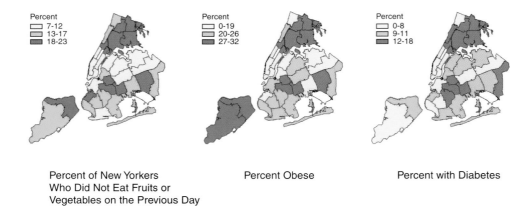

Percent
□ 7-12
▨ 13-17
■ 18-23

Percent
□ 0-19
▨ 20-26
■ 27-32

Percent
□ 0-8
▨ 9-11
■ 12-18

Percent of New Yorkers
Who Did Not Eat Fruits or
Vegetables on the Previous Day

Percent Obese

Percent with Diabetes

FIGURE 2-1 Neighborhoods where fruit and vegetable consumption is low have high rates of obesity and diabetes.
SOURCE: New York Department of Health and Mental Hygiene, 2004 Community Health Survey.

partner from a local university or health department can provide necessary epidemiological or statistical support. Figure 2-1 and Box 2-5 illustrate the use of mapping to assess community health statistics.

2. Involve Constituents

Community involvement is vital to implementing effective childhood obesity prevention efforts. If people feel free to speak and are listened to, they may reveal barriers to healthy eating and physical activity or identify critical community needs of which local government officials and staff are not aware. Local government officials and staff also should consider developing, co-convening, or supporting a community partnership that can help determine needs, prioritize actions, and contribute to advancing community efforts on obesity prevention. Many national youth organizations with local chapters across the country could be helpful, such as the Boys and Girls Clubs, youth sports and recreation leagues, YMCA and YWCA, 4-H clubs, and Boy and Girl Scouts. In addition to or in conjunction with such partnerships, an interagency planning commission can include effective representation of the key local departments and agencies with jurisdiction for ensuring action and fostering sustained efforts. Box 2-6 provides a brief overview of the community engagement and partnership efforts found to be effective in King County, Washington.

Box 2-5
Communicating Community Statistics with Maps

Maps allow local officials to relate characteristics of a community to its geographic layout. Considering that the place where one lives has a significant effect on health, it is helpful to understand and represent data about that place visually. Mapping using geographic information systems has been shown to be a critical tool in performing a community assessment. Maps are an efficient, low-cost way to explain complex statistics associated with particular places, and from a different vantage point than is gained through words. In addition, when seemingly unrelated data are represented spatially, it is often possible to make associations that might otherwise not have been apparent. Maps can highlight farmers' markets, access to food stores, parks, places to walk, public transportation routes, shops, access to health care, and other features that help provide for a healthy community.

When performing an assessment of diet-related diseases, New York City collected data on fruit and vegetable consumption, obesity rates, and diabetes rates and represented those data spatially through maps. Comparison of these maps revealed a clear visual association between the neighborhoods that consumed the fewest fruits and vegetables and those with the highest rates of obesity and diabetes. This information provided a clear target for where the city should direct its Green Cart program, a program that encouraged street vendors to sell low-cost fruits and vegetables. Using maps of the city showing such factors as income, population density, automobile access, and access to fruits and vegetables, the city also developed a map illustrating areas most in need of grocery stores. The Community Farm Alliance performed a similar investigation of Louisville, Kentucky. Through spatially represented data, the organization was able to demonstrate a significant lack of grocery stores in certain areas.

Maps can be used as tools in communicating such data to important stakeholders. The Food Trust in Philadelphia created maps, much like those mentioned previously, indicating the critical areas of the city in need of supermarkets. Showing these maps helped engage public- and private-sector leaders in acting on this issue.

SOURCES: Flournoy, 2009; Karpyn, 2009; Thomases, 2009.

3. Identify Top Policy Priorities

By assessing current food and physical activity environments and involving constituents in determining community needs, local government officials and staff can identify top policy priorities for their community. An assessment of the local environment for obesity prevention will help identify community assets, focus resources, and refine implementation plans.

4. Identify Funding Sources

Sufficient and sustained funding is needed for many new programs and initiatives. However, innovative use of leadership and convening opportunities can further obesity prevention efforts at low or nominal cost. For example, a mayor's leadership, using the bully pulpit of his or her office, is "free" but can positively influence the actions and culture of a community. A county commissioner's support in convening concerned community members or providing support to fledgling coalitions can translate into strategic community actions for a relatively minimal investment. Developing and enacting policies and ordinances, including those that contribute to childhood obesity prevention, is part of the operating costs of local governments. As illustrated in Box 2-7, a potential first step in preventing and

Box 2-7
Organizing to Form a Food Policy Advisory Committee

Access to healthy food for some neighborhoods in New Orleans has long been a problem, even before Hurricane Katrina, but the storm dramatically reduced access in many areas of the city. In 2006, about a year after the storm hit, fewer than half the supermarkets that had been open before the storm were operating. Recognizing the difficulties of accessing healthy foods and the potential to make long-term changes, several community groups began meeting to address the issue. One coalition of groups, Grow New Orleans, led by the New Orleans Food and Farm Network, sought to improve community food security and expand the use of locally produced foods. A second group, the Healthy Eating Coalition, led by Tulane University's Prevention Research Center, was focused on improving access to healthy foods.

The two groups joined forces and, rather than form an autonomous food policy council, decided to work within the context of city government. Advice was sought and received from The Food Trust, an organization that has had substantial success in improving retail food access in Pennsylvania. Discussions began with members of the Special Development Projects and Economic Development Committee, a standing committee of the New Orleans City Council. The initial goal was to receive authorization to form an advisory committee to the City Council, a committee that would be charged with preparing a strategy report on how to improve retail access.

In April 2007, eight organizations—the Tulane Prevention Research Center (PRC), the Second Harvest Food Bank of Greater New Orleans, the Renaissance Project, Steps to a Healthier Louisiana/New Orleans, the Louisiana Public Health Institute, the City of New Orleans Health Department, the New Orleans Food and Farm Network, and The Food Trust—made their case before the Economic Development Committee, which unanimously endorsed the idea. The full City Council approved a resolution authorizing creation of a Food Policy Advisory Committee, and charged it with making recommendations for addressing the lack of access to healthy food in New Orleans. The Council tasked Tulane's Prevention Research Center with empaneling the committee and requested a final report within 8 months.

Key members from each of the local organizations served as a staff for the Food Policy Advisory Committee. The committee itself was made up of 32 leaders from various sectors, including the private retail food sector, both chain and independent grocers; farmers' markets and local agriculture; lending and grant-making institutions; retail suppliers and associations; nonprofit organizations focused on hunger, poverty, children, health, and local food; public health agencies and city government; and academia. Four general meetings were held over the course of several months. An additional three themed meetings focused on the city's planning process, on retail issues, and on regional food and farmers' markets. By the fourth and final general meeting, a list of 10 recommendations had been drafted that summarized the committee's discussions.

continued

In January 2008, a final report based on these recommendations was presented to the City Council. The City Council unanimously adopted a resolution expressing support for the recommendations and approving creation of a task force to develop strategies for their implementation. The task force, formed from the Food Policy Advisory Committee, has helped advance specific strategies for the city, focusing especially on a fresh food retail incentives program. The task force has also met with representatives of the New Orleans Police Department to discuss security for grocery stores and has recommended policies for inclusion in the city's ongoing Master Plan Project. A central purpose of the task force is to maintain momentum and accountability for policy implementation.

SOURCE: Diego Rose, Tulane University, http://www.sph.tulane.edu/PRC/Files/FPAC%20Report%20Final.pdf.

reversing childhood obesity—the creation of a food, physical activity, or health policy council—requires minimal funding and can set the stage for successful prevention efforts.

As discussed earlier, building on the goals and actions of other policy changes can further the obesity prevention agenda. For example, advocating for policies and programs developed to meet goals in a city's sustainability plan (Box 2-1) may provide funding for efforts that meet obesity prevention goals as well. A childhood obesity prevention effort is likely to find broader financial support if it meets the diverse needs of other stakeholders in the community. In addition, it is important to remember that federal nutrition assistance programs—such as the Supplemental Nutrition Assistance Program (SNAP) (formerly the Food Stamp Program), the Special Supplemental Nutrition Program for Women, Infants and Children, the Summer Food Service Program, Afterschool Snacks, and the Child and Adult Care Food Program—are dependable sources of federal funds that provide millions of dollars to communities across the country. These programs can fund healthy meals and snacks—a foundation upon which children's anti-obesity programs can be developed—for example, by providing nutritious meals and related nutrition education to children in summer recreation programs through the Summer Food Service Program, or using farmers' markets (which allow for the use of SNAP benefits in purchasing food) to recruit community members to be involved in broader childhood obesity prevention efforts. Other federal programs (e.g., the Centers for Disease Control and Prevention's Healthy Communities Programs, housing assistance, health care benefits and community health centers, and transportation grants) can provide opportunities for implementing efforts directly relevant to childhood obesity prevention.

Cultivation of funding sources should encompass careful attention to grant opportunities. This includes monitoring federal and state funding that is directly related to obesity prevention or that can help fund projects that meet several local government goals, including childhood obesity prevention. Community and locally based foundations are often a good place to start. Creative thinking is key to fundraising efforts, as the example in Box 2-8 demonstrates. It is often necessary to combine a number of funding streams to achieve an objective, and public–private partnerships may also be fruitful avenues to explore.

Box 2-8
Finding Funding and Resources

The Parks Department in Henderson, Texas, an east Texas county seat of almost 12,000 people, determined there was significant interest among important groups, such as the school board and civic organizations, in an expanded and improved walking and bicycle path network throughout the city. When confronted with the reality of a lack of resources in its budget, the department was able to locate resources from diverse sources. In addition to benefiting from city funds generated by sales taxes, the city learned of a grant from the Texas Parks and Wildlife Department, which provides park development grants to match 50 percent of local contributions. The city also needed access to land on which to build these paths. Instead of securing funding to buy the land, the city coordinated a "land swap" with a private land owner for land near the city's park, in exchange for city-owned land elsewhere in Henderson. Fortunately, the department was able to count this land as an in-kind contribution toward its matched funding grant with the Parks and Wildlife Department. These creative funding solutions have been successful in making it possible to build several miles of paths, which the city intends to be only the beginning of a more extensive network to be completed by 2018.

SOURCE: Barrow, 2009.

5. Think About Program Sustainability

Childhood obesity is a health problem that does not develop in a short period of time, and preventing obesity requires healthy food choices and sustained physical activity throughout one's lifetime. Changes in food and physical activity environments require a culture change, which, while more difficult to accomplish, will have a more lasting impact than short-term promotional programs. The key to sustainability for childhood obesity efforts is, to the extent possible, to make them part of the community infrastructure. Policy changes that are embodied in law in the form of ordinances, regulations and standards, zoning laws, taxes, and the like are more likely to be sustainable. Changes in the built environment—for example, the building or repair of sidewalks or the development of parks and playgrounds—by their very nature are sustainable. Community involvement in identifying, prioritizing, and effecting changes also plays an important role in sustainability because it encourages individuals, families, and organizations to take ownership of the changes and become invested in maintaining them for the long term.

6. Evaluate Programs and Policies

To ensure that obesity prevention initiatives reach the intended populations and have a positive impact, it is important to include provisions for evaluating their reach and effectiveness. Well-conducted evaluations allow policy makers to allocate limited resources to tackling the problem in the most efficient ways for their community. Furthermore, regular evaluation of obesity prevention actions allows local governments to adapt policies to changing demographics of the local population and provide the best use of resources. Information and lessons learned from these efforts can help local governments develop even better programs and policies. Moreover, because evidence is lacking on the effectiveness of many promising childhood obesity prevention strategies, program and policy evaluations add to the knowledge base and allow other communities and program planners to see what does and does not work. In cases where full-scale evaluations are unlikely, requiring the establishment of a system to collect data on program operations makes future research and evaluation possible. Box 2-9 illustrates an innovative way of tracking obesity rates.

Partnering with universities is an excellent way for a local government agency to collect information in the community and monitor and analyze ongoing efforts. For example, Somerville, Massachusetts, partnered with Tufts University to develop and evaluate a comprehensive childhood obesity initiative called Shape Up Somerville (see Box 2-10).

Box 2-9
Using Immunization Registries to Track Obesity Rates

The state of Michigan and San Diego County, California, recently made the decision to use their existing electronic immunization registries as a way to track obesity rates among children. The state and county will add data fields for height and weight to the web-based registry, which will be used to calculate body mass index (BMI), a commonly used measure for defining overweight and obesity. The data gathered from such systems can be extremely valuable in tracking the obesity epidemic and evaluating the effectiveness of ongoing obesity intervention programs, something not currently possible in these jurisdictions.

SOURCE: Altarum Institute, http://www.altarum.org.

CALL TO ACTION

Children need a healthy environment in which to learn, engage, and thrive in a community. Local government can be an integral part of the response to the childhood obesity epidemic. At the local level, government has the authority to authorize and appropriate funds for policies and programs that promote healthy eating and active living. Many existing policies can be amended to increase their health impact. New programs and policies can be formulated based on the best available evidence and examples from across the country. These programs and policies should be chosen based on the needs and characteristics of individual communities. This report highlights a number of programs and policies in the form of case studies; many more such examples of local governments that are translating childhood obesity prevention strategies into action could be cited. Chapters 4 and 5 present the most promising strategies and actions for consideration and evaluation by local governments.

Box 2-10
Comprehensive Obesity Prevention Efforts in an Urban Setting

Shape Up Somerville (SUS) is a city-wide campaign to increase daily physical activity and healthy eating through programming, physical infrastructure improvements, and policy changes. It began as a community-based research study at Tufts University targeting first to third graders. The study demonstrated that city-wide changes could have a positive effect on weight gain among children (Economos et al., 2007). The campaign now targets all segments of the community, including schools, city government, civic organizations, community groups, businesses, and others who live and work in Somerville, Massachusetts—a densely populated, ethnically diverse town of 77,000 located two miles north of Boston. Overall efforts and successes of the program since its inception include the following:

• The Somerville School Food Service Department enhanced the quality and quantity of healthy foods for students.
• Teachers were trained to implement a new health curriculum in class and after school.
• Walking school buses were implemented, crosswalks were repainted, and more crossing guards were hired to encourage walking to school.
• Infrastructure improvements, such as bike lanes and paths, were made.
• Parks were renovated and sites identified for new parks and open space.
• Restaurants increased healthy options or altered portion sizes to become "Shape Up Somerville Approved."

Now, 5 years later, SUS is run by the City of Somerville, led by Mayor Joe Curtatone. The mayor has been a key proponent of the program since its inception. Today, a director and a coordinator work on active and healthy living programs supported by the health department and a task force that is a collaboration of more than 11 initiatives and 25 stakeholders involved in working on various interventions across the city. The task force is steeped in the city and community business cultures. The City of Somerville is working to educate elected officials and community leaders about SUS and is leveraging grant and city funds to maintain permanent SUS staffing positions. SUS has shown that a variety of community-wide changes can help prevent weight gain in young children.

SOURCE: See www.somervillema.gov.

REFERENCES

Baehr, N. 2008. On the frontier against obesity. *Northwest Public Health* Spring/Summer.

Baker, E. L., and J. Porter. 2005. Practicing management and leadership: Creating the information network for public health officials. *Journal of Public Health Management and Practice* 11(5):469–473.

Barrow, M. 2009. City of Henderson, Texas park plan: For a more active, healthy community. Presentation at the IOM Workshop on Childhood Obesity Prevention in Texas, Austin, TX.

Bassett, M. T., T. Dumanovsky, C. Huang, L. D. Silver, C. Young, C. Nonas, T. D. Matte, S. Chideya, and T. R. Frieden. 2008. Purchasing behavior and calorie information at fast-food chains in New York City, 2007. *American Journal of Public Health* 98(8):1457–1459.

Burton, S., E. H. Creyer, J. Kees, and K. Huggins. 2006. Attacking the obesity epidemic: The potential health benefits of providing nutrition information in restaurants. *American Journal of Public Health* 96(9):1669–1675.

Dillon, C., and C. Rowland. 2008. *Rural Obesity—Strategies to Support Rural Counties in Building Capacity*. Washington, DC: NACo (National Association of Counties).

Duffey, K. 2007. Differential associations of fast-food and restaurant food consumption with 3-y change in body mass index: The coronary artery risk development in young adults (CARDIA) study. *American Journal of Clinical Nutrition* 85:201–208.

Economos, C. D., R. R. Hyatt, J. P. Goldberg, A. Must, E. N. Naumova, J. J. Collins, and M. E. Nelson. 2007. A community intervention reduces BMI z-score in children: Shape up Somerville first year results. *Obesity* 15(5):1325–1336.

ERS (Economic Research Service). 2008. *Diet Quality and Food Consumption: Food Away From Home*. July 2008. http://www.ers.usda.gov/Briefing/DietQuality/FAFH.htm (accessed August 4, 2009).

Flournoy, R. 2009. Research and action to improve community environments and reduce childhood obesity. Presentation at the IOM Community Perspectives on Obesity Prevention in Children Workshop, Washington, DC.

Flournoy, R., and S. Treuhaft. 2005. *Healthy Food, Healthy communities: Improving Access and Opportunities Through Food Retailing*. Oakland, CA: Policylink and The California Endowment.

Frank, L. D., M. A. Andresen, and T. L. Schmid. 2004. Obesity relationships with community design, physical activity, and time spent in cars. *American Journal of Preventive Medicine* 27(2):87–96.

HHS and USDA (U.S. Department of Health and Human Services and U.S. Department of Agriculture). 2005. *Dietary Guidelines for Americans 2005*. http://www.healthierus.gov/dietaryguidelines (accessed February 25, 2009).

IOM (Institute of Medicine). 2005. *Preventing Childhood Obesity: Health in the Balance.* Washington, DC: The National Academies Press.

IOM. 2007. *Progress in Preventing Childhood Obesity: How Do We Measure Up?* Washington, DC: The National Academies Press.

Karpyn, A. 2009. What level of evidence is needed to inform policy makers? Presentation at the IOM Community Perspectives on Obesity Prevention in Children Workshop, Washington, DC.

Lopez, R. P., and H. P. Hynes. 2006. Obesity, physical activity, and the urban environment: Public health research needs. *Environmental Health: A Global Access Science Source 5.*

New York City Department of Health and Mental Hygiene. 2004. *2004 Community Health Survey.* https://a816-healthpsi.nyc.gov/epiquery/EpiQuery/ (accessed August 5, 2009).

Patterson, P. D., C. G. Moore, J. C. Probst, and J. A. Shinogle. 2004. Obesity and physical inactivity in rural America. *Journal of Rural Health* 20(2):151–159.

Thomases, B. 2009. Food policy in New York City. Presentation at the IOM Community Perspectives on Obesity Prevention in Children Workshop, Washington, DC.

Thompson, O. M., C. Ballew, K. Resnicow, A. Must, L. G. Bandini, H. Cyr, and W. H. Dietz. 2004. Food purchased away from home as a predictor of change in BMI z-score among girls. *International Journal of Obesity* 28(2):282–289.

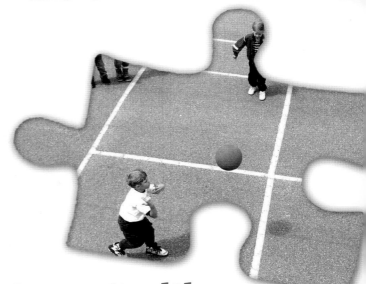

3
Creating Equal Opportunities for Healthy Weight

VIEWING LOCAL GOVERNMENT DECISIONS THROUGH A HEALTH EQUITY LENS

There is a growing national awareness of the major role social, economic, and environmental factors can play in determining the health of individuals and populations. Unequal exposure to positive social, economic, and environmental influences can result in health differences, viewed more properly as inequities, among groups of people. For example, lower-income neighborhoods tend to have environments that are unlikely to encourage or provide access to opportunities for healthy eating and adequate physical activity (Day, 2006).

These neighborhoods are less likely to have the grocery store options or the park and playground facilities found in higher-income neighborhoods (Black and Macinko, 2008; Booth et al., 2005; Kumanyika and Grier, 2006). Additionally, their streets are more likely to be unsafe and difficult to navigate for walkers and cyclists, with fewer walking and bike paths, and their playgrounds are often unsafe. Analyses of the availability of high-calorie, low-nutrient foods and beverages, and the prevalence of advertising, show higher levels in lower-income neighborhoods (Black and Macinko, 2008; Kumanyika and Grier, 2006; Yancey et al., 2009). On the other hand, the availability of nutritious foods, and social marketing on the value and attractiveness of nutritious foods, are less likely in these neighborhoods. Children that are born, grow up, live, work, and age in these environments are more likely to be obese than children from more affluent communities. They are also more likely to suffer from the chronic diseases associated with obesity. Unless changes are made in the social, economic, and environmental factors affecting many children's lives, these seemingly intransigent health problems are likely to continue.

The Institute of Medicine (IOM) report *The Future of the Public's Health in the 21st Century* (IOM, 2003, p. 4) states, "It is unreasonable to expect that people will change their behavior easily when so many forces in the social, cultural, and physical environment conspire against such change." This view is echoed by researchers studying the effect of the social environment on physical activity: "Advising individuals to be more physically active without considering social norms for activity, resources, and opportunities for engaging in physical activity, and environmental constraints such as crime, traffic, and unpleasant surroundings, is unlikely to produce behavior change" (McNeill et al., 2006, p. 1012). Conversely, changing people's environments to provide equal access to factors that determine health will enable them to better control their health and its determinants, make healthier choices, and thereby improve their health.

The charge to local governments, then, is to work with community leaders, members and others to eliminate the inequities outlined above—that is, to create health equity. Many people nationwide at the local, state, and federal levels are working to define this concept and identify ways of applying it to policy, planning, and service delivery. One such definition has been developed by the Centers for Disease Control and Prevention's (CDC's) Health Equity Workgroup: "Health equity is the fair distribution of health determinants, outcomes, and resources within and between segments of the population, regardless of social standing" (CDC, 2007).

Just as glasses with 3-D lenses allow movie audiences to see three-dimensional images that they could not see unaided, looking at communities and their members' health status through the lens of health equity can help policy makers understand the health impacts of such factors as racism, poverty, residential segregation, poor housing, lack of access to quality education, and limited access to health care. Using the health equity lens can also suggest the actions needed to achieve optimal health and health justice. The new perspective provided by seeing through a health equity lens allows local government officials to reframe their viewpoint. Thus, for example, instead of simply noting that a lower-income child eats few fruits and vegetables and does not engage in sufficient physical activity, local government officials can be encouraged to question the equity of distribution of supermarkets, the adequacy of transportation, the safety of neighborhoods, and the availability of parks and recreation opportunities in the context of residential segregation, high rates of unemployment, and an absence of social capital.

This new perspective can point policy makers in the right direction to pursue policies and actions that can reverse the situation in communities with disproportionately high rates of obesity and remove barriers to health equity and good health. Some of the actions local governments can take to make these changes happen are listed below. (Chapters 4 and 5, respectively, outline more specific actions that can be taken to promote healthful eating and physical activity.)

- Improve coordination among agencies and organizations whose activities address determinants of health in such areas as education, housing, planning, agriculture, employment, and economic development.
- Engage with communities in planning and implementing actions to improve health and health equity.
- Find ways to increase the availability of healthy, affordable food in underserved communities and reduce access to unhealthy foods.
- Create a built environment that encourages walking, cycling, and other physical activity.
- Consider cultural barriers that keep lower-income, minority, and immigrant populations from purchasing healthier foods or seeking opportunities for physical activity.
- Work with community partners to identify and build upon cultural assets, such as dance traditions or gardening for groups with a rich farming heritage.

Finally, it is important to recognize that many decisions made by local governments that appear unrelated to childhood obesity actually may have a significant effect. For example, decisions about employee income, education, public assistance, housing assistance, affordable housing plans, transportation, health insurance, commercial development, community involvement in government and decision making, and community policing, to name a few, may have positive or negative impacts on the prevalence of childhood obesity overall and especially among those who are most vulnerable.

Viewing local government decision making through a health equity lens is fundamental to preventing childhood obesity and promoting health equity. This is a matter of ethics and fairness, but it is also a practical necessity because of the financial and human costs associated with obesity. Efforts aimed at preventing childhood obesity should target those areas of the community where the problem is greatest and where social, economic, and environmental factors appear to promote obesity and act as barriers to its prevention. As policy makers and community partners review the strategies and action steps offered in this report, they should focus on those actions that are most likely to lessen health disparities related to childhood obesity and to bring the community's children and their families closer to a state of health equity.

REFERENCES

Black, J. L., and J. Macinko. 2008. Neighborhoods and obesity. *Nutrition Reviews* 66(1):2–20.

Booth, K. M., M. M. Pinkston, and W. S. C. Poston. 2005. Obesity and the built environment. *Journal of the American Dietetic Association* 105(Suppl. 5):S110–S117.

CDC (Centers for Disease Control and Prevention). 2007 (unpublished). *Health Equity Working Group*. Atlanta, GA: CDC.

Day, K. 2006. Active living and social justice: Planning for physical activity in low-income, black, and Latino communities. *Journal of the American Planning Association* 72(1):88–99.

IOM (Institute of Medicine). 2000. *Promoting Health: Intervention Strategies from Social and Behavioral Research*. Washington, DC: National Academy Press.

Kumanyika, S., and S. Grier. 2006. Targeting interventions for ethnic minority and low-income populations. *Future of Children* 16(1):187–207.

McNeill, L. H., M. W. Kreuter, and S. V. Subramanian. 2006. Social environment and physical activity: A review of concepts and evidence. *Social Science and Medicine* 63(4):1011–1022.

Yancey, A. K., B. L. Cole, R. Brown, J. D. Williams, A. Hillier, R. S. Kline, M. Ashe, S. A. Grier, D. Backman, and W. J. McCarthy. 2009. A cross-sectional prevalence study of ethnically targeted and general audience outdoor obesity-related advertising. *The Milbank Quarterly* 87(1):155–184.

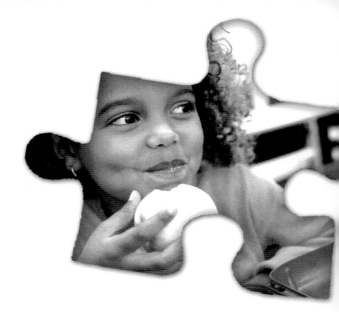

4

Actions for Healthy Eating

The food and physical activity choices made every day affect short- and long-term health and are directly related to weight outcomes. Eating right and being physically active may reduce the risk for heart disease, high blood pressure, diabetes, osteoporosis, certain cancers, and being overweight or obese (HHS and USDA, 2005). These diseases and conditions impact the individual and his or her quality of life and are associated with increasing health care costs that place a burden on the government and businesses. Childhood provides the opportunity to establish a solid foundation that can lead to healthy lifelong eating patterns (IOM, 2005). Prevention of childhood obesity is essential to the promotion of a healthier and more productive society (IOM, 2005). In addition, many diet-related chronic diseases have their origins during childhood and adolescence.

Major changes in the nation's food system and food and eating environments have occurred in recent decades, driven by technological advances; U.S. food and agricultural policies; population growth; and economic, social, and lifestyle changes (Story et al., 2008). Food is now readily available and accessible in many settings throughout the day. The current U.S. food supply contains a large amount of energy-dense foods, many of which consist of refined grains and foods high in fats and/or sugars and low in nutrients. Many of these foods are often available in increasingly large portion sizes at relatively low prices (Story et al., 2008). Americans are also eating out more often and consuming more calories away from home than ever before (Keystone Center, 2006). Moreover, families are eating fewer meals together (Neumark-Sztainer et al., 2003). In addition, the school food environment is radically different than it was a few decades ago, with many schools now offering and promoting high-calorie, low-nutrition foods throughout the school day (Fox et al., 2009). Food marketing aimed at children using multiple channels, such as digital media, has drastically increased as well (IOM, 2006). Finally, an exodus of grocery stores and an influx of fast-food restaurants in lower-income urban areas have contributed to income and racial/ethnic disparities in access to healthier foods (IOM, 2005).

Together, these environmental changes have influenced what, where, and how much Americans eat and have played a large role in the current obesity epidemic. As recommended in the Institute of Medicine (IOM) report *Preventing Childhood Obesity: Health in the Balance*, childhood obesity prevention should be public health in action at its broadest and most inclusive level and a national health priority (IOM, 2005). To be effective, obesity prevention efforts should use public health population-based approaches, including policy and environmental changes that affect large numbers of people. Solving the problem will require the efforts of many stakeholders, including those in the public and private sectors, working together for change.

WHAT IS MEANT BY HEALTHY EATING AND HEALTHY FOODS?

In developing working definitions for *healthy eating* and *healthy foods*, the committee looked to the 2005 Dietary Guidelines for Americans (HHS and USDA, 2005). These guidelines, which are revised every five years and are based on the latest scientific evidence, provide information and advice for choosing a nutritious diet, maintaining a healthy weight, and achieving adequate exercise. The guidelines include 16 key recommendations that focus on food and diet (see Box 4-1). The 2005 guidelines recommend that all healthy Americans aged 2 and older consume a variety of nutrient-dense foods and beverages within and among the basic food groups and limit the intake of saturated and *trans* fats, cholesterol, added sugars, and alcohol. Nutrient-dense foods are foods that provide substantial amounts of vitamins, minerals, and other health-promoting components, such as fiber, for relatively few calories. Foods that are low in nutrient density supply calories but no or small amounts of vitamins, minerals, and health-promoting components (HHS and USDA, 2005). The greater the consumption of foods and beverages that are low in nutrient density and high in fats and sugars, the more difficult it is to achieve energy balance (the balance between calories consumed and calories burned through physical activity and bodily processes) and still meet nutrient needs. The lack of energy balance can lead to unhealthy weight gain. Selecting foods that are consistent with the guidelines (i.e., fruits, vegetables,

Box 4-1
Recommendations of the Dietary Guidelines for Healthy Eating

Adequate Nutrients Within Calorie Needs
- Consume a variety of nutrient-dense foods and beverages within and among the basic food groups while choosing foods that limit the intake of saturated and *trans* fats, cholesterol, added sugars, salt, and alcohol.
- Meet recommended intakes within energy needs by adopting a balanced eating pattern, such as the U.S. Department of Agriculture (USDA) Food Guide or the Dietary Approaches to Stop Hypertension (DASH) Eating Plan.

Weight Management
- To maintain body weight in a healthy range, balance calories from foods and beverages with calories expended.
- To prevent gradual weight gain over time, make small decreases in food and beverage calories and increase physical activity.

Food Groups to Encourage
- Consume a sufficient amount of fruits and vegetables while staying within energy needs. Two cups of fruit and 2½ cups of vegetables per day are recommended for a reference 2,000-calorie intake, with higher or lower amounts depending on the calorie level.
- Choose a variety of fruits and vegetables each day. In particular, select from all five vegetable subgroups (dark green, orange, legumes, starchy vegetables, and other vegetables) several times a week.
- Consume 3 or more ounce-equivalents of whole-grain products per day, with the rest of the recommended grains coming from enriched or whole-grain products. In general, at least half the grains should come from whole grains.
- Consume 3 cups per day of fat-free or low-fat milk or equivalent milk products.

Fats
- Consume less than 10 percent of calories from saturated fatty acids and less than 300 mg/day of cholesterol, and keep *trans* fatty acid consumption as low as possible.
- Keep total fat intake between 20 to 35 percent of calories, with most fats coming from sources of polyunsaturated and monounsaturated fatty acids, such as fish, nuts, and vegetable oils.
- When selecting and preparing meat, poultry, dry beans, and milk or milk products, make choices that are lean, low-fat, or fat-free.
- Limit intake of fats and oils high in saturated and/or *trans* fatty acids, and choose products low in such fats and oils.

continued

Box 4-1 Continued

Carbohydrates
- Choose fiber-rich fruits, vegetables, and whole grains often.
- Choose and prepare foods and beverages with little added sugars or caloric sweeteners, such as amounts suggested by the USDA Food Guide and the DASH Eating Plan.
- Reduce the incidence of dental caries by practicing good oral hygiene and consuming sugar- and starch-containing foods and beverages less frequently.

Sodium And Potassium
- Consume less than 2,300 mg (approximately 1 teaspoon of salt) of sodium per day.
- Choose and prepare foods with little salt. At the same time, consume potassium-rich foods, such as fruits and vegetables.

SOURCE: HHS and USDA, 2005.

whole grains, and low- or non-fat dairy products) and watching portion sizes is the best way to maintain a healthy weight while meeting nutrient needs.

In accordance with the Dietary Guidelines, in this report *healthy eating* refers to eating the types and amounts of foods, nutrients, and calories recommended in those guidelines. *Healthy foods* refers to fruits and vegetables with minimal or no added sugar, fat, or salt; fat-free or low-fat dairy products; whole grains; and lean meats. Healthy foods are also rich in health-promoting nutrients needed for overall wellness, such as fiber, vitamins, and minerals. These working definitions are tailored to the childhood obesity problem and the need to address dietary excesses and inadequacies associated with the current eating patterns of children and youth.

There is no widely accepted definition of *calorie-dense, nutrient-poor foods*, nor is there consensus on which foods should be included in this category. The 2005 Dietary Guidelines for Americans introduced the concept of "discretionary" calories—the extra calories that are consumed during a day as added fat and/or sugars after enough healthy foods have been consumed to meet caloric and nutrient needs. Most discretionary calorie allowances are very small, between 100 and 300 calories, especially for those who are not physically active. This report uses the term *calorie-dense, nutrient-poor foods* to refer to those foods and beverages that contribute few vitamins and minerals to the diet but contain substantial amounts of fat and/or sugar and are high in calories. Consumption of these foods, such as sugar-sweetened beverages, candy, and chips, may contribute to excess caloric intake and unwanted weight gain in children. Moreover, these foods may replace more nutritious foods, leading to decreased intake of some micronutrients (Kant, 2003; Swinburn et al., 2004).

CREATING A HEALTHY EATING ENVIRONMENT

Although food consumption is ultimately a matter of individual choice, local food environments influence the choices made by children, families, and community members. In the 2001 *Surgeon General's Call to Action to Prevent and Decrease Overweight and Obesity,* former U.S. Surgeon General David Satcher stated, "Individual behavior change can occur only in a supportive environment with accessible and affordable healthy food choices and opportunities for regular physical activity" (HHS, 2001). Effective obesity prevention policy and practices that address changes to the environment can help individuals take responsibility for improving their food choices. The failure of individual-based nutrition and physical activity efforts can be explained, in part, because the environments where they have been implemented are not conducive to healthful choices (Booth et al., 2001). The healthy choice must also be the easy choice.

A *healthy eating environment* is one in which families have access to supermarkets or other places where they can obtain affordable healthy foods such as fruits and vegetables; healthy food is available and easy to identify in restaurants and public buildings; lower-income community members are informed about and participate in federal nutrition programs, such as the Supplemental Nutrition Assistance Program (SNAP, formerly called the Food Stamp Program); women feel supported and comfortable in breastfeeding; and there are ample water fountains in public places. This chapter reviews ways in which local governments can create an environment with these basic characteristics that supports healthy eating.

DISPARITIES IN ACCESS TO HEALTHY FOODS

As discussed in Chapter 3, the healthy choice is often the more difficult choice in some neighborhoods. Lower-income and minority neighborhoods and communities suffer disproportionately high rates of preventable, diet-related diseases, including obesity (Ford and Dzewaltowski, 2008; Morland and Evenson, 2009), and inequalities in access to affordable, healthy, and nutritious food contribute to these disparities. Access to healthy food in many lower-income urban and rural areas is often lacking and is of particular concern because of the negative impact on dietary intake and obesity among a vulnerable population. Lower-income areas are less likely to have access to supermarkets and grocery stores that carry healthy foods compared with predominantly white, middle- and higher-income neighborhoods (Baker et al., 2006; Franco et al., 2008; Morland et al., 2002). Many stores in lower-income neighborhoods are smaller with a limited number of products and fewer healthy items such as fruits and vegetables, low-fat or non-fat dairy products, and whole grains. Public transportation to supermarkets is often lacking as well (Morland et al., 2002). Research suggests that neighborhood residents who have better access to supermarkets and limited access to convenience stores tend to have healthier diets and lower levels of obesity (Lopez, 2007; Morland et al., 2006; Powell et al., 2007). A poor food environment in lower-income areas may be exacerbated by an abundance of fast-food restaurants serving high-calorie, high-fat meals at relatively low prices (Lewis et al., 2005). The availability of fast-food restaurants and calorie-dense foods is greater in lower-income and minority neighborhoods (Baker et al., 2006; Larson et al., 2009).

Few studies have evaluated strategies for reducing disparities by improving access to healthy, affordable foods and reducing access to high-calorie, low-nutrition foods. Several strategies and actions have been proposed to attract supermarkets to underserved neighborhoods, improve the availability of healthy foods such as fruits, vegetables and whole grain products, and reduce access to calorie-dense foods in fast food establishments and restaurants. As discussed in Chapter 3, to address childhood obesity, local governments should consider giving priority to neighborhoods and communities that lack access to healthy foods and/or have a relative excess of unhealthy foods. Rates of obesity and obesity-related illnesses tend to be higher in these communities (Morland and Evenson, 2009).

THE ROLE OF LOCAL GOVERNMENTS IN PROMOTING HEALTHY EATING

Local governments can have a strong and direct impact on people's health and well-being and are well positioned to make positive changes in food environments in communities. Local governments can provide strategic leadership, such as providing improved access to healthy foods in lower-income areas, using zoning laws to change local food environments, requiring menu labeling in restaurants, serving as a catalyst for community change by offering healthier foods at government facilities, developing the infrastructure necessary for obesity prevention policies and programs to be implemented and evaluated at the local level, and communicating the importance of healthy eating and obesity prevention to community members. Local governments can and should provide opportunities to change the community food environment to positively influence individual food choices by making the healthy choice the easy choice.

Local governments have a role to play in both increasing access to healthy foods *and* reducing access to unhealthy foods. To date, and as reflected in this report, there are more access-enhancing strategies than those that might reduce access to unhealthy foods. However, local governments should also focus on strategies that reduce access to unhealthy foods, as these potentially may have more of an impact in reducing obesity than increasing access to healthy foods. For example, restricting access to sugar-sweetened beverages in after-school community programs may have more of an impact on reducing the consumption of excess calories and weight gain in youth than opening a farmers' market once a week for five months or starting a community garden. Finally, while some initiatives may not have a direct impact on healthy eating behaviors, they may strengthen ties among diverse and important community stakeholders. Broad-based coalitions or organizational strengths developed through such activities can facilitate effective advocacy for subsequent initiatives that have more impact but are more difficult to implement.

The healthy eating strategies and action steps recommended by the committee for local governments' consideration are organized around three goals:

1. Improve access to and consumption of healthy, safe, and affordable foods.
2. Reduce access to and consumption of calorie-dense, nutrient-poor foods.
3. Raise awareness about the importance of healthy eating to prevent childhood obesity.

This list of goals and the strategies and action steps discussed under each are not prioritized, but, as stated in the introduction, certain action steps are bolded as being most promising. Local community leaders, members, and policy makers will be in the best position to decide which strategies and action steps will be most feasible and appropriate for the needs and circumstances of their community. The decision will be based largely on such factors as resources, priorities, leadership, and demographics. Following are the goals, strategies, and action steps related to healthy eating.

GOAL 1: IMPROVE ACCESS TO AND CONSUMPTION OF HEALTHY, SAFE, AND AFFORDABLE FOOD

Strategy 1: Retail Outlets

Increase community access to healthy foods through supermarkets, grocery stores, and convenience/corner stores.

Rationale

People cannot consume a healthy diet unless healthy foods are available, affordable, and convenient. Research suggests that neighborhood residents who have better access to supermarkets and grocery stores tend to have healthier diets and lower levels of obesity (Larson et al., 2009; Lopez, 2007; Morland and Evenson, 2009; Story et al., 2008). Access to supermarkets and grocery stores can also lead to increased fruit and vegetable intake (Casagrande et al., 2009; Rose and Richards, 2004). The presence of small food store and corner stores also influences diet (Bodor et al., 2008). Residents of lower-income, minority, and rural neighborhoods are most likely to have poor access to supermarkets and other venues with healthy foods (Black and Macinko, 2008; Larson et al., 2009; Story et al., 2008). These individuals are more likely to have a high body mass index (BMI) (Inagami et al., 2006). Evidence suggests that using urban planning land use policies to increase access to supermarkets can decrease BMI in adolescents (Powell et al., 2007).

The committee recognizes the complexities of some of the following action steps; some may require more time, resources, or support than others. It is important to consider groundwork that may make these action steps easier to implement. For example, to attract supermarkets to underserved communities, local governments may need to create policies designed to help businesses and others navigate the complex development process.

Action Steps

- **Create incentive programs to attract supermarkets and grocery stores to underserved neighborhoods (e.g., tax credits, grant and loan programs, small business/economic development programs, and other economic incentives).**
- Realign bus routes or provide other transportation, such as mobile community vans or shuttles to ensure that residents can access supermarkets or grocery stores easily and affordably through public transportation.

- Create incentive programs to enable current small food store owners in underserved areas to carry healthier, affordable food items (e.g., grants or loans to purchase refrigeration equipment to store fruits, vegetables, and fat-free/low-fat dairy; free publicity; a city awards program; or linkages to wholesale distributors).
- Use zoning regulations to enable healthy food providers to locate in underserved neighborhoods (e.g., "as of right" and "conditional use permits").
- Enhance accessibility to grocery stores through public safety efforts, such as better outdoor lighting and police patrolling.

Strategy 2: Restaurants

Improve the availability and identification of healthful foods in restaurants.

Rationale

Americans are eating away from home more than ever before (French et al., 2001). Foods from away-from-home sources are higher in calories and fat compared with at-home foods (French et al., 2001). Eating out more frequently, especially at fast-food restaurants, is associated with obesity (Duffey, 2007; Rosenheck, 2008). Without clear, easy-to-use nutrition information at the point of ordering, it is difficult to make informed choices at restaurants. Preliminary findings from localities that have instituted menu labeling show that consumers may choose more healthy options when they are informed about the nutritional quality of offerings (Bassett et al., 2008; Harnack and French, 2008; Technomic Inc., 2009).

Action Steps

- **Require menu labeling in chain restaurants to provide consumers with calorie information on in-store menus and menu boards.**
- Encourage non-chain restaurants to provide consumers with calorie information on in-store menus and menu boards.
- Offer incentives (e.g., recognition or endorsement) for restaurants that promote healthier options (for example, by increasing the offerings of healthier foods, serving age-appropriate portion sizes, or making the default standard options healthy—i.e., apples or carrots instead of French fries, and non-fat milk instead of soda in "kids' meals").

Strategy 3: Community Food Access

Promote efforts to provide fruits and vegetables in a variety of settings, such as farmers' markets, farm stands, mobile markets, community gardens, and youth-focused gardens.

Rationale

Increasing the availability of fruits and vegetables is an important means of improving the quality of the diet. Fruit and vegetables are relatively low in calories and, because of their high fiber and water content, can increase satiety and reduce overall calorie intake (Rolls et al., 2004). Substituting fruits and vegetables for higher calorie foods such as those high in fat and added sugars can be a component of a successful obesity prevention strategy (CDC, 2007). Evidence suggests that promoting farmers' markets can increase fruit and vegetable intake (Herman et al., 2008; Kropf et al., 2007). Community gardens and garden-based nutrition intervention programs may also have the potential to promote increased fruit and vegetable intake (Alaimo et al., 2008) and may increase willingness to taste fruits and vegetables among youth (Robinson-O'Brien et al., 2009).

Action Steps

- Encourage farmers markets to accept Special Supplemental Nutrition Program for Women, Infants and Children (WIC) food package vouchers and WIC Farmers' Market Nutrition Program coupons; and encourage and make it possible for farmers' markets to accept Supplemental Nutrition Assistance Program (or SNAP, formerly the Food Stamp Program) and WIC Program Electronic Benefit Transfer (EBT) cards by allocating funding for equipment that uses electronic methods of payment.
- Improve funding for outreach, education, and transportation to encourage use of farmers' markets and farm stands by residents of lower-income neighborhoods, and by WIC and SNAP recipients.
- Introduce or modify land use policies/zoning regulations to promote, expand and protect potential sites for community gardens and farmers' markets, such as vacant city-owned land or unused parking lots.
- Develop community-based group activities (e.g., community kitchens) that link procurement of affordable, healthy food with improving skills in purchasing and preparing food.

Strategy 4: Public Programs and Worksites

Ensure that publicly run entities such as after-school programs, child care facilities, recreation centers, and local government worksites implement policies and practices to promote healthy foods and beverages and reduce or eliminate the availability of calorie-dense, nutrient-poor foods.

Rationale

National studies consistently show that the diets of children and adolescents do not meet national recommendations for good health, are contributing to overweight and obesity, and are placing youth at risk for serious health consequences (HHS and USDA, 2005; IOM, 2005). Places where children gather and spend much of their time should contribute to a healthful food environment. Since many children spend time in after-school programs, child care, and recreation centers, making sure that the food served in these settings is healthy could help to improve their diets. Research suggests that the nutritional quality of meals and snacks in child care settings can be poor and activity levels may be inadequate (Ball et al., 2008; Padget and Briley, 2005; Story et al., 2006). Furthermore, children model the behavior of adults (Pearson et al., 2009). Ensuring that publicly run entities mandate strong nutrition standards in facilities and programs that serve children and adults would imply that healthy eating is an important issue. Local government agencies can serve as leaders and role models by adopting policies and practices that promote healthy food choices in public places.

Action Steps

- **Mandate and implement strong nutrition standards for foods and beverages available in government-run or regulated after-school programs, recreation centers, parks, and child care facilities (which includes limiting access to calorie-dense, nutrient-poor foods).**
- Ensure that local government agencies that operate cafeterias and vending options have strong nutrition standards in place wherever foods and beverages are sold or available.
- Provide incentives or subsidies to government-run or -regulated programs and localities that provide healthy foods at competitive prices and limit calorie-dense, nutrient-poor foods (e.g., after-school programs that provide

fruits or vegetables every day, and eliminate calorie-dense, nutrient-poor foods in vending machines or as part of the program).

Strategy 5: Government Nutrition Programs

Increase participation in federal, state, and local government nutrition assistance programs (e.g., WIC, School Breakfast and Lunch Programs, the Child and Adult Care Food Program, the Afterschool Snacks Program, the Summer Food Service Program, SNAP).

Rationale

Nutrition assistance programs provide children and lower-income people access to food for a healthful diet. They are not associated with increased weight in children or adults (Hofferth and Curtin, 2005; Ver Ploeg, 2009; Ver Ploeg et al., 2008). In fact, recent research from the School Nutrition Dietary Assessment Study-III showed that children who participated in the School Breakfast Program had a lower likelihood of overweight and obesity (Gleason and Dodd, 2009). Other research suggests similar associations with School Lunch, SNAP, and the WIC program (Bitler and Currie, 2004; Jones et al., 2003). Furthermore, recent revisions to the WIC food package increased the amount of whole grains, fruits, and vegetables participants receive, making it even easier for lower-income mothers and children to eat the healthy foods recommended by the Dietary Guidelines.

Action Steps

- Put policies in place that require government-run and -regulated agencies responsible for administering nutrition assistance programs to collaborate across agencies and programs to increase enrollment and participation in these programs (i.e., WIC agencies should ensure that those who are eligible are also participating in SNAP, etc.).
- Ensure that child care and after-school program licensing agencies encourage utilization of the nutrition assistance programs and increase nutrition program enrollment (CACFP, the Afterschool Snack Program, and the Summer Food Service Program).

Strategy 6: Breastfeeding

Encourage breastfeeding and promote breastfeeding-friendly communities.

Rationale

Breastfeeding has multiple health benefits for infants and mothers. Research shows that the longer a child breastfeeds, the less likely he or she is to be overweight. (Arenz et al., 2004; Moreno and Rodriguez, 2007). But despite national recommendations to increase breastfeeding initiation and duration rates, many barriers make it difficult for mothers to continue breastfeeding. Local governments can implement policies and programs that make it easier for mothers to breastfeed. For example, mothers that give birth in "baby-friendly hospitals" that practice the United Nations Children's Fund/World Health Organization (UNICEF/WHO) ten steps to successful breastfeeding, part of the Baby-Friendly Hospital Initiative USA, are more likely to exclusively breastfeed (Declercq et al., 2009).

Action Steps

- Adopt practices in city and county hospitals that are consistent with the Baby-Friendly Hospital Initiative USA (UNICEF/WHO). This initiative promotes, protects, and supports breastfeeding through ten steps to successful breastfeeding for hospitals.
- Permit breastfeeding in public places and rescind any laws or regulations that discourage or do not allow breastfeeding in public places and encourage the creation of lactation rooms in public places.
- Develop incentive programs to encourage government agencies to ensure breastfeeding-friendly worksites, including providing lactation rooms.
- Allocate funding to WIC clinics to acquire breast pumps to loan to participants.

Strategy 7: Drinking Water Access

Increase access to free, safe drinking water in public places to encourage water consumption in place of sugar-sweetened beverages.

Sugar-sweetened beverage intake is considered an important contributing factor to obesity in childhood (James and Kerr, 2005; Malik et al., 2009; Moreno and Rodriguez, 2007; Vartanian et al., 2007). Replacing sugar-sweetened beverages with water is associated with reductions in total energy intake for children and adolescents (Wang et al., 2009). Installing water fountains in public places and facilities can increase water intake and prevent and reduce overweight and obesity (Muckelbauer et al., 2009).

Action Steps

- Require that plain water be available in local government-operated and administered outdoor areas and other public places and facilities.
- **Adopt building codes to require access to, and maintenance of, fresh drinking water fountains (e.g., public restroom codes).**

GOAL 2: REDUCE ACCESS TO AND CONSUMPTION OF CALORIE-DENSE, NUTRIENT-POOR FOODS

Strategy 8: Policies and Ordinances

Implement fiscal policies and local ordinances to discourage the consumption of calorie-dense, nutrient-poor foods and beverages (e.g., taxes, incentives, land use and zoning regulations).

Rationale

Increasing access and consumption of healthy foods alone will not necessarily reduce excess caloric intake and body weight. Reducing access to and consumption of calorie-dense, nutrient-poor foods is also needed to decrease excess calories and help prevent obesity in children. These foods are often high in refined grains, added fats, and sugars and tend to be inexpensive and convenient (Monsivais and Drewnowski, 2007). Children today have near constant access to calorie-dense, nutrient-poor foods and beverages. Fast food restaurants and other purveyors of inexpensive, unhealthy food are often densely located in lower-income, urban neighborhoods (Baker et al., 2006). They are also often located near schools, which can increase obesity rates (Currie et al., 2009). Moreover, advertising of fast-food restaurants can also affect obesity rates (Chou et al., 2008). Taxing calorie-dense, nutrient-poor foods is one method that might decrease consumption (Brownell and Frieden, 2009; Congressional Budget Office, 2008). Zoning and land use policies that regulate fast food restaurants may affect consumption as well (Ashe et al., 2003; Paquin, 2008). It is important to point out that there are local and state legal issues that need to be considered in any restriction of advertising efforts or imposition of food and beverage taxes. In addition, jurisdiction over these issues can vary from community to community.

Action Steps

- **Implement a tax strategy to discourage consumption of foods and beverages that have minimal nutritional value, such as sugar-sweetened beverages.**
- Adopt land use and zoning policies that restrict fast food establishments near school grounds and public playgrounds.
- Implement local ordinances to restrict mobile vending of calorie-dense, nutrient-poor foods near schools and public playgrounds.
- Implement zoning designed to limit the density of fast food establishments in residential communities.
- Eliminate advertising and marketing of calorie-dense, nutrient-poor foods and beverages near school grounds and public places frequently visited by youths.
- Create incentive and recognition programs to encourage grocery stores and convenience stores to reduce point-of-sale marketing of calorie-dense, nutrient-poor foods (i.e., promote "candy-free" check out aisles).

GOAL 3: RAISE AWARENESS ABOUT THE IMPORTANCE OF HEALTHY EATING TO PREVENT CHILDHOOD OBESITY

Strategy 9: Media and Social Marketing

Promote media and social marketing campaigns on healthy eating and childhood obesity prevention.

Rationale

Media can be a key element to increase awareness and motivation and can be used to promote healthy eating, portion size awareness, eating fewer calorie-dense, nutrient-poor foods and to raise awareness of weight as a health issue.

High-frequency television and radio advertising, as well as signage, may stimulate improvements in attitudes toward a healthy diet (Beaudoin et al., 2007). A media approach may even cause a community to alter its dietary habits (Reger et al., 1999). Depending on the resources available, and the purpose of the campaign, both local development of campaigns and the adoption of national message campaigns may be useful. In keeping with the report's focus on changes that local governments can make to improve the food and physical activity environments of children, it is important to point out that media and social marketing campaigns can improve these local environments by highlighting the reasons for improving children's food and physical activity environments; and engaging the public in taking advantage of new resources in their environment such as farmers' markets, new grocery stores, healthier choices at local businesses, etc.

Action Steps

- **Develop media campaigns, utilizing multiple channels (print, radio, Internet, television, social networking, and other promotional materials) to promote healthy eating (and active living) using consistent messages.**
- Design a media campaign that establishes community access to healthy foods as a health equity issue and reframes obesity as a consequence of environmental inequities and not just the result of poor personal choices.
- Develop counter-advertising media approaches against unhealthy products to reach youth as has been used in the tobacco and alcohol prevention fields.

REFERENCES

Alaimo, K., E. Packnett, R. A. Miles, and D. J. Kruger. 2008. Fruit and vegetable intake among urban community gardeners. *Journal of Nutrition Education and Behavior* 40(2):94–101.

Arenz, S., R. Ruckerl, B. Koletzko, and R. Von Kries. 2004. Breast-feeding and childhood obesity: A systematic review. *International Journal of Obesity* 28(10):1247–1256.

Ashe, M., D. Jernigan, R. Kline, and R. Galaz. 2003. Land use planning and the control of alcohol, tobacco, firearms, and fast food restaurants. *American Journal of Public Health* 93(9):1404–1408.

Baker, E. A., M. Schootman, E. Barnidge, and C. Kelly. 2006. The role of race and poverty in access to foods that enable individuals to adhere to dietary guidelines. *Preventing Chronic Disease [electronic resource]* 3(3).

Ball, S. C., S. E. Benjamin, and D. S. Ward. 2008. Dietary intakes in North Carolina child-care centers: Are children meeting current recommendations? *Journal of the American Dietetic Association* 108(4):718–721.

Bassett, M. T., T. Dumanovsky, C. Huang, L. D. Silver, C. Young, C. Nonas, T. D. Matte, S. Chideya, and T. R. Frieden. 2008. Purchasing behavior and calorie information at fast-food chains in New York City, 2007. *American Journal of Public Health* 98(8):1457–1459.

Beaudoin, C. E., C. Fernandez, J. L. Wall, and T. A. Farley. 2007. Promoting healthy eating and physical activity. Short-term effects of a mass media campaign. *American Journal of Preventive Medicine* 32(3):217–223.

Bitler, M. P., and J. Currie. 2004. Medicaid at birth, WIC take up, and children's outcomes. *RAND Labor and Population working paper series.*

Black, J. L., and J. Macinko. 2008. Neighborhoods and obesity. *Nutrition Reviews* 66(1):2–20.

Bodor, J. N., D. Rose, T. A. Farley, C. Swalm, and S. K. Scott. 2008. Neighbourhood fruit and vegetable availability and consumption: The role of small food stores in an urban environment. *Public Health Nutrition* 11(4):413–420.

Booth, S. L., J. F. Sallis, C. Ritenbaugh, J. O. Hill, L. L. Birch, L. D. Frank, K. Glanz, D. A. Himmelgreen, M. Mudd, B. M. Popkin, K. A. Rickard, S. St. Jeor, and N. P. Hays. 2001. Environmental and societal factors affect food choice and physical activity: Rationale, influences, and leverage points. *Nutrition Reviews* 59(3 II).

Brownell, K., and T. R. Frieden. 2009. Ounces of prevention—the public policy case for taxes on sugared beverages. *New England Journal of Medicine* 360(18):1805–1917.

Casagrande, S. S., M. C. Whitt-Glover, K. J. Lancaster, A. M. Odoms-Young, and T. L. Gary. 2009. Built environment and health behaviors among African Americans. A systematic review. *American Journal of Preventive Medicine* 36(2):174–181.

CDC (Centers for Disease Control and Prevention). 2007. Can eating fruits and vegetables help people to manage their weight? *Research to Practice Series, No. 1.* http://www.cdc.gov/nccdphp/dnpa/nutrition/pdf/rtp_practitioner_10_07.pdf (accessed March 4, 2009).

Chou, S. Y., I. Rashad, and M. Grossman. 2008. Fast-food restaurant advertising on television and its influence on childhood obesity. *Journal of Law and Economics* 51(4):599–618.

Congressional Budget Office. 2008. *Health Care.* Washington, DC: Congressional Budget Office.

Currie, J., S. DellaVigna, E. Moretti, and V. Pathania. 2009. *The Effect of Fast Food Restaurants on Obesity.* Cambridge, MA: National Bureau of Economic Research.

Declercq, E., M. Labbok, C. Sakala, and M. O'Hara. 2009. Hospital practices and women's likelihood of fulfilling their intention to exclusively breastfeed. *American Journal of Public Health* 99(5):929–935.

Duffey, K. 2007. Differential associations of fast-food and restaurant food consumption with 3-y change in body mass index: The coronary artery risk development in young adults (CARDIA) study. *American Journal of Clinical Nutrition* 85:201–208.

Ford, P. B., and D. A. Dzewaltowski. 2008. Disparities in obesity prevalence due to variation in the retail food environment: Three testable hypotheses. *Nutrition Reviews* 66(4):216–228.

Fox, M. K., A. Gordon, R. Nogales, and A. Wilson. 2009. Availability and consumption of competitive foods in U.S. public schools. *Journal of the American Dietetic Association* 109(2):S57–S66.

Franco, M., A. V. Diez Roux, T. A. Glass, B. Caballero, and F. L. Brancati. 2008. Neighborhood characteristics and availability of healthy foods in Baltimore. *American Journal of Preventive Medicine* 35(6):561–567.

French, S. A., M. Story, and R. W. Jeffery. 2001. Environmental influences on eating and physical activity. In *Annual Review of Public Health*.

Gleason, P. M., and A. H. Dodd. 2009. School breakfast program but not school lunch program participation is associated with lower body mass index. *Journal of the American Dietetic Association* 109(2):S118–S128.

Harnack, L. J., and S. A. French. 2008. Effect of point-of-purchase calorie labeling on restaurant and cafeteria food choices: A review of the literature. *International Journal of Behavioral Nutrition and Physical Activity* 5.

Herman, D. R., G. G. Harrison, A. A. Afifi, and E. Jenks. 2008. Effect of a targeted subsidy on intake of fruits and vegetables among low-income women in the special supplemental nutrition program for women, infants, and children. *American Journal of Public Health* 98(1):98–105.

HHS (U.S. Department of Health and Human Services). 2001. *The Surgeon General's Call to Action to Prevent and Decrease Overweight and Obesity*. http://www.surgeongeneral. gov/topics/obesity/calltoaction/CalltoAction.pdf (accessed May 12, 2009).

HHS and USDA (U.S. Department of Agriculture). 2005. *Dietary Guidelines for Americans 2005*. http://www.healthierus.gov/dietaryguidelines (accessed February 25, 2009).

Hofferth, S. L., and S. Curtin. 2005. Poverty, food programs, and childhood obesity. *Journal of Policy Analysis and Management* 24(4):703–726.

Inagami, S., D. A. Cohen, B. K. Finch, and S. M. Asch. 2006. You are where you shop. Grocery store locations, weight, and neighborhoods. *American Journal of Preventive Medicine* 31(1):10–17.

IOM (Institute of Medicine). 2005. *Preventing Childhood Obesity: Health in the Balance*. Washington, DC: The National Academies Press.

IOM. 2006. *Food Marketing to Children and Youth: Threat or Opportunity?* Washington, DC: The National Academies Press.

James, J., and D. Kerr. 2005. Prevention of childhood obesity by reducing soft drinks. *International Journal of Obesity* 29(Suppl. 2):S54–S57.

Jones, S. J., L. Jahns, B. A. Laraia, and B. Haughton. 2003. Lower risk of overweight in school-aged food insecure girls who participate in food assistance: Results from the panel study of income dynamics child development supplement. *Archives of Pediatrics and Adolescent Medicine* 157(8):780–784.

Kant, A. K. 2003. Reported consumption of low-nutrient-density foods by American children and adolescents: Nutritional and health correlates, NHANES III, 1988 to 1994. *Archives of Pediatrics and Adolescent Medicine* 157(8):789–796.

Keystone Center. 2006. *The Keystone Forum on Away from-Home Foods: Opportunities for Preventing Weight gain and Obesity.* Washington, DC: Keystone Center.

Kropf, M. L., D. H. Holben, J. P. Holcomb, Jr., and H. Anderson. 2007. Food security status and produce intake and behaviors of special supplemental nutrition program for women, infants, and children and farmers' market nutrition program participants. *Journal of the American Dietetic Association* 107(11):1903–1908.

Larson, N. I., M. T. Story, and M. C. Nelson. 2009. Neighborhood environments. Disparities in access to healthy foods in the U.S. *American Journal of Preventive Medicine* 36(1):74–81.

Lewis, L. B., D. C. Sloane, L. M. Nascimento, A. L. Diamant, J. J. Guinyard, A. K. Yancey, and G. Flynn. 2005. African Americans' access to healthy food options in south Los Angeles restaurants. *American Journal of Public Health* 95(4):668–673.

Lopez, R. P. 2007. Neighborhood risk factors for obesity. *Obesity* 15(8):2111–2119.

Malik, V. S., W. C. Willett, and F. B. Hu. 2009. Sugar-sweetened beverages and BMI in children and adolescents: Reanalyses of a meta-analysis. *American Journal of Clinical Nutrition* 89(1):438–439.

Monsivais, P., and A. Drewnowski. 2007. The rising cost of low-energy-density foods. *Journal of the American Dietetic Association* 107(12):2071–2076.

Moreno, L. A., and G. Rodriguez. 2007. Dietary risk factors for development of childhood obesity. *Current Opinion in Clinical Nutrition and Metabolic Care* 10(3):336–341.

Morland, K. B., and K. R. Evenson. 2009. Obesity prevalence and the local food environment. *Health and Place* 15(2):491–495.

Morland, K., S. Wing, A. Diez Roux, and C. Poole. 2002. Neighborhood characteristics associated with the location of food stores and food service places. *American Journal of Preventive Medicine* 22(1):23–29.

Morland, K., A. V. Diez Roux, and S. Wing. 2006. Supermarkets, other food stores, and obesity: The atherosclerosis risk in communities study. *American Journal of Preventive Medicine* 30(4):333–339.

Muckelbauer, R., L. Libuda, K. Clausen, A. M. Toschke, T. Reinehr, and M. Kersting. 2009. Promotion and provision of drinking water in schools for overweight prevention: Randomized, controlled cluster trial. *Pediatrics* 123(4):e661–e667.

Neumark-Sztainer, D., P. J. Hannan, M. Story, J. Croll, and C. Perry. 2003. Family meal patterns: Associations with sociodemographic characteristics and improved dietary intake among adolescents. *Journal of the American Dietetic Association* 103(3):317–322.

Padget, A., and M. E. Briley. 2005. Dietary intakes at child-care centers in central Texas fail to meet food guide pyramid recommendations. *Journal of the American Dietetic Association* 105(5):790–793.

Paquin, S. 2008. Zoning and classification of uses for restaurants and commercial food establishments: A measure of urban planning to reduce the epidemic of obesity. *Canadian Journal of Urban Research* 17(Suppl. 1):48–62.

Pearson, N., S. J. Biddle, and T. Gorely. 2009. Family correlates of fruit and vegetable consumption in children and adolescents: A systematic review. *Public Health Nutrition* 12(2):267–283.

Powell, L. M., M. C. Auld, F. J. Chaloupka, P. M. O'Malley, and L. D. Johnston. 2007. Associations between access to food stores and adolescent body mass index. *American Journal of Preventive Medicine* 33(Suppl. 4):S301–S307.

Reger, B., M. G. Wootan, and S. Booth-Butterfield. 1999. Using mass media to promote healthy eating: A community-based demonstration project. *Preventive Medicine* 29(5):414–421.

Robinson-O'Brien, R., M. Story, and S. Heim. 2009. Impact of garden-based youth nutrition intervention programs: A review. *Journal of the American Dietetic Association* 109(2):273–280.

Rolls, B. J., J. A. Ello-Martin, and B. C. Tohill. 2004. What can intervention studies tell us about the relationship between fruit and vegetable consumption and weight management? *Nutrition Reviews* 62(1):1–17.

Rose, D., and R. Richards. 2004. Food store access and household fruit and vegetable use among participants in the U.S. food stamp program. *Public Health Nutrition* 7(8):1081–1088.

Rosenheck, R. 2008. Fast food consumption and increased caloric intake: A systematic review of a trajectory towards weight gain and obesity risk. *Obesity Reviews* 9(6):535–547.

Story, M., K. M. Kaphingst, and S. French. 2006. The role of child care settings in obesity prevention. *Future of Children* 16(1):143–168.

Story, M., K. M. Kaphingst, R. Robinson-O'Brien, and K. Glanz. 2008. Creating healthy food and eating environments: Policy and environmental approaches. *Annual Review of Public Health* 29:253–272.

Swinburn, B. A., I. Caterson, J. C. Seidell, and W. P. T. James. 2004. Diet, nutrition and the prevention of excess weight gain and obesity. *Public Health Nutrition* 7(1A):123–146.

Technomic Inc. 2009. *Consumer Reaction to Calorie Disclosure on Menus/Menu Boards in New York City.* Chicago, IL: Technomic, Inc.

UNICEF/WHO (United Nations Children's Fund/World Health Organization). *Baby friendly hospital initiative.* http://www.babyfriendlyusa.org/eng/index.html (accessed June 10, 2009).

Vartanian, L. R., M. B. Schwartz, and K. D. Brownell. 2007. Effects of soft drink consumption on nutrition and health: A systematic review and meta-analysis. *American Journal of Public Health* 97(4):667–675.

Ver Ploeg, M. 2009. *WIC and the Battle Against Childhood Overweight.* Washington, DC: USDA Economic Research Service.

Ver Ploeg, M., L. Mancino, B. H. Lin, and J. Guthrie. 2008. U.S. food assistance programs and trends in children's weight. *International Journal of Pediatric Obesity* 3(1):22–30.

Wang, Y. C., D. S. Ludwig, K. Sonneville, and S. L. Gortmaker. 2009. Impact of change in sweetened caloric beverage consumption on energy intake among children and adolescents. *Archives of Pediatrics and Adolescent Medicine* 163(4):336–343.

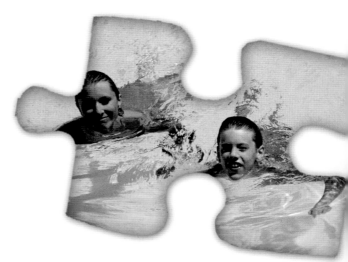

5

Actions for Increasing Physical Activity

Research shows that a sedentary lifestyle is a predictor of overweight and obesity (Must and Tybor, 2005). Physical activity is critical not only for optimal weight, but also for physical and cognitive development in childhood. Current recommendations are for children to engage in physical activity at least 60 minutes per day (HHS and USDA, 2008); this includes any physical activity accumulated throughout the day, such as playing, walking to school, and exercise. However, many children are not that active. A 2002 Centers for Disease Control and Prevention (CDC) survey found that 61.5 percent of children aged 9–13 did not participate in any organized physical activity during their nonschool hours and that 22.6 percent did not engage in any free-time physical activity (CDC, 2003). These findings reflect marked increases during the past several decades in sedentary activities of daily living among both children and adults (Brownson et al., 2005). This more sedentary lifestyle is the result of increased reliance on technology and labor-saving devices, such as use of automobiles rather than walking or biking, attributable in part to community designs that favor this mode of transport; use of washing machines and dishwashers in the household; less physical activity in the workplace because of computers and automated equipment; increased use of television and computers for entertainment and leisure activities; and use of elevators and escalators rather than stairs. In addition, increased concern about crime has reduced the likelihood of outdoor playing; and decreased walking and bicycling and increased driving in response to community design that favors cars (Goran and Treuth, 2001). These activities reduce the need for daily physical activity or make it more difficult to be physically active.

CREATING A HEALTHY ENVIRONMENT FOR PHYSICAL ACTIVITY

Aspects of what researchers and planners call the "built environment" are important determinants of physical activity for both children and adults and therefore of rates of childhood obesity (Black and Macinko, 2008; Booth et al., 2005). The built environment encompasses all of the man-made elements of the physical environment, including buildings, infrastructure, and other physical elements created or modified by people (e.g., sidewalks, streets, trails, bicycle lanes, parks, playgrounds), as well as the functional use, arrangement in space, and aesthetic qualities of these elements (e.g., zoning, neighborhood design, mixed-use development) (IOM, 2005). Handy (2005) categorizes these elements as follows:

- Land use—the location and intensity of activities, including residential, commercial, and institutional activities, and the design and arrangement of the buildings and sites that house them.
- Transportation systems—the physical layout and design of roads, sidewalks, bike paths, and other transportation infrastructure, and their function and appearance.

The "social environment" is just as important to physical activity. It includes such elements as family, friends, place of employment, home, culture, socioeconomic status, and neighborhood. The social environment also encompasses neighborhood reputation, defined by perceived safety and social nuisances, as well as social support and social capital (Black and Macinko, 2008). For example, parental modeling of and support for participation in physical activity (e.g., by providing transportation and purchasing equipment) has been associated with higher levels of physical activity in children (Hoefer et al., 2001; Sallis et al., 2000).

However, the environment in which some children live often makes it difficult to engage in physical activity. Many neighborhoods lack open space, parks, recreational facilities, or sports fields. Neighborhood features that encourage physical activity are consistently associated with decreased weight. Among these factors, mixed land use, access to fitness facilities, and neighborhood "walkability" have all been linked to higher levels of physical activity and lower body weight (Black and Macinko, 2008). These are all aspects of the built environment.

The built environment's influence on childhood obesity is determined by its effect on physical activity levels and also, as the previous chapter explains, its effect on healthy eating. It can promote or deter physical activity, such as organized active recreation, active commuting, and unstructured play. Various elements of the built environment affect different types of physical activity in a number of ways. For example, the distance from home to school or to the soccer field is a key factor in whether children walk or bicycle to these places rather than being driven (Handy and Tal, 2008; Kerr et al., 2006; McDonald, 2007). Safety along the route, whether from traffic or "stranger danger," is also important (Carver et al., 2008; Davison and Lawson, 2006). The design of neighborhoods influences outdoor play outside of the school day. Access to parks and other safe places to play, for example, is associated with more frequent outdoor play (Davison and Lawson, 2006; Mota et al., 2005). If there are safe and appealing opportunities to walk, bicycle, play, or otherwise move outdoors, thus creating an environment that promotes physical activity, children are likely to engage in more physical activity.

DISPARITIES IN THE BUILT AND SOCIAL ENVIRONMENTS

A number of the elements that constitute beneficial built and social environments—such as good sidewalks, low-speed streets, attractive greenspaces, nearby trails, easily accessible recreation centers, people visible walking or playing outdoors, and low crime rates—often are characteristic of communities with higher socioeconomic status (SES). Lower-SES communities often must deal with the negative aspects of the environment, such as busy through streets, poor-quality bicycle and pedestrian infrastructure, dilapidated parks and playgrounds, and crime, that deter physical activity (Black and Macinko, 2008; Booth et al., 2005). In addition to low SES, a high concentration of minority populations is a predictor for such disparities. Neighborhoods with large Hispanic and African American populations, for example, are less likely to have public parks and private recreation facilities (Gordon-Larsen et al., 2006). Lack of availability of facilities that enable and promote physical activity may, in part, explain the lower levels of activity observed among low-SES and minority communities (Powell et al., 2006), as may hazardous conditions such as crime (Seefeldt et al., 2002). Therefore, as discussed in Chapter 3, local governments should make low-SES and minority neighborhoods a priority when implementing the action steps outlined in this chapter to address disparities in the built and social environments.

THE ROLE OF LOCAL GOVERNMENTS IN PROMOTING PHYSICAL ACTIVITY

Local governments have an important role to play in supporting and promoting physical activity, in large part through their influence on the built environment, but through other means as well. Local governments, particularly cities, have significant power over the form of the built environment (Handy and Clifton, 2007). Through general plans and zoning codes, cities and other local government entities make decisions on land use policies and plan and design street layouts and locations, including requirements for sidewalks and allowable street widths. They also own and maintain neighborhood parks and playgrounds, and in many cases operate and maintain other recreational facilities. They can set requirements for developers to provide sidewalks, walking and biking trails, and greenspace in new developments, as well as invest public money in enhance existing areas. Through these actions, local governments create—or restrict—opportunities for physical activity for children.

Local governments can support physical activity in other ways as well. Parks and recreation departments, for example, often run sports leagues or offer dance, gymnastics, or other active classes. Many cities have worked with school districts to promote walking and bicycling to school through Safe Routes to School programs and related initiatives. More general efforts to improve traffic safety and enforce traffic laws make streets safer for children to walk, bicycle, and play. Such programs help ensure that children take advantage of opportunities afforded by the built environment and compensate for its deficiencies. Furthermore, local governments can provide support and resources to local organizations that want to create healthy environments.

The physical activity strategies and actions recommended by the committee for consideration by local governments are organized around three goals:

1.   Encourage physical activity.
2.   Decrease sedentary behavior.
3.   Raise awareness about the importance of increasing physical activity.

For each goal, several strategies and action steps are provided, as well as examples of how some communities have implemented these actions. This list of goals and the strategies and action steps discussed under each are not prioritized, but, as stated in the introduction, certain action steps are bolded as being most promising. Local community leaders, members, and policy makers will be in the best position to decide which strategies and action steps will be most feasible and appropriate for the needs and circumstances of their community. The decision will be based largely on such factors as resources, priorities, leadership, and demographics. Following are the goals, strategies, and action steps related to physical activity.

GOAL 1: ENCOURAGE PHYSICAL ACTIVITY

Strategy 1: Built Environment

Encourage walking and bicycling for transportation and recreation through improvements in the built environment.

Rationale

Walking and bicycling, whether for transportation or recreation, are important sources of physical activity for children as well as adults. Walking, in particular, has been described by health researchers as near perfect exercise (Lee and Buchner, 2008). The built environment has a significant effect on walking and bicycling. Deficiencies in walking and bicycling infrastructure and streets designed for vehicles create barriers to walking and bicycling. Community residents are less likely to walk or bicycle for transportation or recreation if streets do not include sidewalks and safe crossings (Badland and Schofield, 2005; Davison and Lawson, 2006; Saelens et al., 2003). Residents of lower-income neighborhoods are more likely to face challenges posed by streets and sidewalks in disrepair, missing or blocked sidewalks and poorly marked crossings. Excessively wide streets encourage speeding, thereby increasing risks to pedestrians and bicyclists. Traffic volume and speed are negatively associated with children's participation in physical activity (Davison and Lawson, 2006). Many rural roads, where speed limits are high, lack shoulders that can accommodate a pedestrian or cyclist. Land use patterns also deter walking and bicycling. Community residents are less likely to walk or bicycle for transportation if distances to destinations such as schools, recreation, and shopping are far (Saelens and Handy, 2008).

Improvements to these elements of the built environment can encourage walking and bicycling. Research shows that older, traditional neighborhoods with a mix of uses and well-connected street networks support physical activity as residents walk or ride their bicycle to nearby destinations (Badland and Schofield, 2005; Frank et al., 2004). Building and maintaining sidewalks and safe street crossings appears to hold some promise in promoting physical activity in neighborhoods (Lee and Moudon, 2008). Sidewalks may even affect obesity (Booth et al., 2005). Infrastructure improvements in the vicinity of schools can increase the number of children who walk and bicycle (Boarnet et al., 2005). Less experienced pedestrians and bicyclists may feel more comfortable on trails and paths separated from vehicle traffic. Community-scale and street-scale urban design and land use policies and practices; proximity of residential areas to stores, jobs, schools and recreation areas; continuity and connectivity of sidewalks and streets; and aesthetic and safety aspects of the physical environment can all have an effect on physical activity rates (CDC, 2006b). Local governments can make these improvements through many different actions, some applied to new development and some to retrofitting existing areas, as noted in the boxes below. While a comprehensive approach is most effective, it's important to note that simple changes, even a new coat of paint on a crosswalk, can have an impact on physical activity in a community.

Action Steps

- Adopt a pedestrian and bicycle master plan to develop a long-term vision for walking and bicycling in the community and guide implementation.
- **Plan, build, and maintain a network of sidewalks and street crossings that creates a safe and comfortable walking environment and that connects to schools, parks, and other destinations.**

Ways in Which Some Local Governments Have Implemented This Action Step

- Establish a sidewalk maintenance program to insure that existing sidewalks are kept in a good state of repair. [retrofit]*
- Develop a program to fill gaps in the sidewalk network, especially on routes near schools, transit stops, and retail. [retrofit]
- Establish an intersection/pedestrian crossing retrofit program to make it easier for pedestrians to cross streets safely. [retrofit]
- Revise subdivision ordinances or other codes to require sidewalks and safe pedestrian crossings in all new developments. [new]
- Revise city/county codes to require short, well-connected blocks or a minimum number of intersections to provide direct connections between destinations. [new]

---

* Retrofit: Modification of infrastructure and facilities in existing areas of the community rather than the provision of infrastructure and facilities in new areas of development.

- Plan, build, and retrofit streets so as to reduce vehicle speeds, accommodate bicyclists, and improve the walking environment.

Ways in Which Some Local Governments Have Implemented This Action Step

- Establish a traffic calming program, especially in neighborhoods negatively impacted by speeding, to slow traffic and improve safety and comfort for all users. [retrofit]
- Reduce the number of lanes through a "road diet" program on streets with four or more lanes where traffic volumes can be managed in two or three lanes. [retrofit]
- Revise design standards to ensure that new streets are properly sized for moderate vehicle speeds and are consistent with a Complete Streets Policy. [new]
- Establish a program to create slow, shared street environments, known as "home zones," for residential streets with low traffic volumes. [new and retrofit]

- Plan, build, and maintain a well-connected network of off-street trails and paths for pedestrians and bicyclists.

Ways in Which Some Local Governments Have Implemented This Action Step

- Look for opportunities to build or expand path/trail networks, e.g., rails-to-trails projects. [retrofit]
- Amend the land development code to require developers to dedicate land for and/or build trails and paths that link to the existing network of trails and paths. [new]

- Increase destinations within walking and bicycling distance.

Ways in Which Some Local Governments Have Implemented This Action Step

- Adopt zoning codes that support higher density and mixed-use development around neighborhood centers and transit stations. [new and retrofit]
- Establish programs and incentives that encourage developers to fill in older, underused parts of the community with housing, supermarkets, and other services. [retrofit]
- Modify land use plans and development codes to require that new developments have mixed-use, higher density community centers with schools, parks, and retail within walking distance of housing. [new]

- Collaborate with school districts and developers to build new schools in locations central to residential areas and away from heavily trafficked roads.

Strategy 2: Programs for Walking and Biking

Promote programs that support walking and bicycling for transportation and recreation.

Rationale

Local governments can encourage residents to be more physically active by establishing programs that increase safety, provide education, and otherwise facilitate walking and bicycling. Perceived safety has a significant effect on walking for both children and adults (Carver et al., 2008; Cleland et al., 2008; Weir et al., 2006). Crime has an effect on physical activity as well (Ferreira et al., 2007; Gordon-Larsen et al., 2000). Providing children with a safe environment in which they can walk or bicycle to school can increase physical activity. Children who walk or bicycle to school have higher daily levels of physical activity and better cardiovascular fitness than do children who do not actively commute to school (Davison et al., 2008). Riding a bicycle at least two or more days during the week is associated with a decreased likelihood of being overweight during childhood (Dudas and Crocetti, 2008). Access to bicycles and safety equipment are necessary precursors to safe bicycling. Transit users have higher levels of physical activity owing to walking to transit stops (Zheng, 2008). Programs that support walking and bicycling often require partnerships with other organizations or agencies.

Action Steps

- **Adopt community policing strategies that improve safety and security of streets, especially in higher crime neighborhoods.** *
- **Collaborate with schools to develop and implement a Safe Routes to School program to increase the number of children safely walking and bicycling to schools.**
- Improve access to bicycles, helmets, and related equipment for lower-income families, for example, through subsidies or repair programs.
- Promote increased transit use through reduced fares for children, families, and students, and improved service to schools, parks, recreation centers, and other family destinations.
- Implement a traffic enforcement program to improve safety for pedestrians and bicyclists.

Strategy 3: Recreational Physical Activity

Promote other forms of recreational physical activity.

Rationale

Recreational activities such as playing on a playground or shooting hoops are an important source of physical activity for children. Children who spend more time outdoors have higher levels of physical activity (Sallis et al., 2000). Access to neighborhood parks may increase levels of physical activity and reduce time spent in sedentary behaviors at home (Floriani and Kennedy, 2008; Kaczynskl and Henderson, 2008). Children are less likely to engage in recreational physical activity if parks or playgrounds are unavailable, in disrepair, or are not accessible by safe routes (Grow et al., 2008; Kaczynskyl and Henderson, 2008). This is especially true in higher-density lower-income neighborhoods that were built before

*Two action steps on community policing were combined for the most promising 12 action steps list.

the establishment of park acreage requirements, where more residents are living in closer proximity to one another, and where public budgets may be insufficient to cover maintenance needs (Day, 2006). Participation in athletic activities is another way for children to increase physical activity and possibly lower body weight (Bélanger et al., 2009; Elkins et al., 2004; Weintraub et al., 2008), as is increasing access to recreation facilities (Baker et al., 2008; Sallis and Glanz, 2009).

Action Steps

- **Build and maintain parks and playgrounds that are safe and attractive for playing, and in close proximity to residential areas.**

Ways in Which Some Local Governments Have Implemented This Action Step

- Adopt a Parks Master Plan to develop a long-term vision for parks and help prioritize implementation. [new and retrofit]
- Develop or revise park design standards to establish minimums for amount of park land per resident, types of play facilities for children, etc. [new and retrofit]
- Establish a program to maintain and upgrade existing parks and playgrounds. [retrofit]
- Establish a program to identify small vacant parcels that can be converted to pocket parks, especially in densely populated, older neighborhoods. [retrofit]
- Amend the land development code to require developers to dedicate land for and/or build parks and playgrounds. [new]
- Consider innovative playground equipment that is weather-proof and vandalism-resistant and permits a range of individual and group fitness activities. [new and retrofit]

- **Adopt community policing strategies that improve safety and security for park use, especially in higher crime neighborhoods.***

---

*Two action steps on community policing were combined for the most promising 12 action steps list.

- Improve access to public and private recreational facilities in communities with limited recreational options through reduced costs, increased operating hours, and development of culturally appropriate activities.
- Create after-school activity programs, e.g., dance classes, city-sponsored sports, supervised play, and other publicly or privately supported active recreation.
- **Collaborate with school districts and other organizations to establish joint use of facilities agreements allowing playing fields, playgrounds, and recreation centers to be used by community residents when schools are closed; if necessary, adopt regulatory and legislative policies to address liability issues that might block implementation.**
- Create and promote youth athletic leagues and increase access to fields, with special emphasis on income and gender equity.
- Build and provide incentives to build recreation centers in neighborhoods.

Strategy 4: Routine Physical Activity

Promote policies that build physical activity into daily routines.

Rationale

Building physical activity into daily routines makes physical activity automatic by making the active choice the default choice (Yancey, 2007). This is especially important because individuals most in need of increased physical activity are the least likely to choose to engage in physical activity. Approaches such as point-of-decision prompts to encourage use of stairs can increase physical activity in places frequented by children (CDC, 2006b). Changes in institutional practices and the built environment that structurally integrate physical activity into routines can increase automatic physical activity and are critical for widespread activity-promoting social norm change (Bower et al., 2008; Donnelly et al., 2009; IOM, 2006; Lara et al., 2008).

Action Steps

- **Institute regulatory policies mandating minimum play space, physical equipment, and duration of play in preschool, after-school, and child care programs.**

- Develop worksite policies and practices that build physical activity into routines (for example, exercise breaks at a certain time of day and in meetings or walking meetings). Target worksites with high percentages of youth employees and government-run and -regulated worksites.
- Create incentives for remote parking and drop-off zones and/or disincentives for nearby parking and drop-off zones at schools, public facilities, shopping malls, and other destinations.
- Improve stairway access and appeal, especially in places frequented by children.

GOAL 2: DECREASE SEDENTARY BEHAVIOR

Strategy 5: Screen Time

Promote policies that reduce sedentary screen time.

Rationale

Every day, 8- to 18-year-olds spend an average of four hours watching TV, videos, DVDs, and prerecorded shows; just over one hour on the computer; and about 50 minutes playing video games (Roberts et al., 2005). Research shows that reducing screen time reduces the likelihood of being overweight (Jackson et al., 2009). According the American Academy of Pediatrics, children should limit total screen time to 2 hours or less per day (Bar-On et al., 2001). Children that meet this recommendation and meet physical activity recommendations are least likely to be overweight (Laurson et al., 2008). Behavioral interventions to reduce screen time can have a positive effect on obesity (CDC, 2006a).

Action Steps

- Adopt regulatory policies limiting screen time in preschool and after-school programs.

GOAL 3: RAISE AWARENESS ABOUT THE IMPORTANCE OF INCREASING PHYSICAL ACTIVITY

Strategy 6: Media and Social Marketing

Develop a social marketing campaign that emphasizes the multiple benefits for children and families of sustained physical activity.

Rationale

Media can be a key element to increase awareness and motivation and can be used to promote physical activity, decrease sedentary activity and to raise awareness of weight as a health issue. Evidence suggests that community-wide campaigns to increase physical activity can be effective (CDC, 2006b). High-frequency television and radio advertising, as well as signage may stimulate improvements in attitudes toward walking behavior (Beaudoin et al., 2007). The national VERB campaign is an example of a social marketing campaign that positively influenced physical activity in children. After 2 years, children in communities that received a high dose of VERB campaign advertising and promotional activities reported higher awareness and understanding of VERB, greater self-efficacy, more sessions of physical activity per week, and were more active on the day before being surveyed than children who received the average national dose (Berkowitz et al., 2008). Depending on the resources available, and the purpose of the campaign, both local development of campaigns and the adoption of national message campaigns may be useful. In keeping with the focus on changes that local governments can make to improve the food and physical activity environments of children, it is important to point out that media and social marketing campaigns can improve these environments by focusing on the reasons for improving children's food and physical activity environments; and engaging the public in taking advantage of new resources in their environment such as recreation centers, playgrounds, walking paths, etc.

Action Steps

- Develop media campaigns, utilizing multiple channels (print, radio, Internet, television, other promotional materials) to promote physical activity using consistent messages.

- Design a media campaign that establishes physical activity as a health equity issue and reframes obesity as a consequence of environmental inequities and not just the result of poor personal choices.
- Develop counter-advertising media approaches against sedentary activity to reach youth as has been done in the tobacco and alcohol prevention fields.

REFERENCES

Badland, H., and G. Schofield. 2005. Transport, urban design, and physical activity: An evidence-based update. *Transportation Research Part D: Transport and Environment* 10(3):177–196.

Baker, E. A., M. Schootman, C. Kelly, and E. Barnidge. 2008. Do recreational resources contribute to physical activity? *Journal of Physical Activity and Health* 5(2):252–261.

Bar-On, M. E., D. D. Broughton, S. Buttross, S. Corrigan, A. Gedissman, M. R. Gonzalez De Rivas, M. Rich, D. L. Shifrin, M. Brody, B. Wilcox, M. Hogan, H. J. Holroyd, L. Reid, S. N. Sherry, V. Strasburger, and J. Stone. 2001. Children, adolescents, and television. *Pediatrics* 107(2):423–426.

Beaudoin, C. E., C. Fernandez, J. L. Wall, and T. A. Farley. 2007. Promoting healthy eating and physical activity. Short-term effects of a mass media campaign. *American Journal of Preventive Medicine* 32(3):217–223.

Bélanger, M., K. Gray-Donald, J. O'Loughlin, G. Paradis, J. Hutcheon, K. Maximova, and J. Hanley. 2009. Participation in organised sports does not slow declines in physical activity during adolescence. *International Journal of Behavioral Nutrition and Physical Activity* 6:22.

Berkowitz, J. M., M. Huhman, and M. J. Nolin. 2008. Did augmenting the VERB campaign advertising in select communities have an effect on awareness, attitudes, and physical activity? *American Journal of Preventive Medicine* 34(Suppl. 6):S257–S266.

Black, J. L., and J. Macinko. 2008. Neighborhoods and obesity. *Nutrition Reviews* 66(1):2–20.

Boarnet, M. G., K. Day, C. Anderson, T. McMillan, and M. Alfonzo. 2005. California's safe routes to school program: Impacts on walking, bicycling, and pedestrian safety. *Journal of the American Planning Association* 71(3):301–317.

Booth, K. M., M. M. Pinkston, and W. S. C. Poston. 2005. Obesity and the built environment. *Journal of the American Dietetic Association* 105(Suppl. 5):S110–S117.

Bower, J. K., D. P. Hales, D. F. Tate, D. A. Rubin, S. E. Benjamin, and D. S. Ward. 2008. The childcare environment and children's physical activity. *American Journal of Preventive Medicine* 34(1):23–29.

Brownson, R. C., T. K. Boehmer, and D. A. Luke. 2005. Declining rates of physical activity in the United States: What are the contributors? In *Annual Review of Public Health* 26:421–443.

Carver, A., A. Timperio, and D. Crawford. 2008. Playing it safe: The influence of neighbourhood safety on children's physical activity a review. *Health and Place* 14(2):217–227.

CDC (Centers for Disease Control and Prevention). 2003. Physical activity levels among children aged 9–13 years—United States, 2002. *Morbidity and Mortality Weekly Report* 52(33):785–788.

CDC. 2006a. *Guide to Community Preventive Services: Obesity Prevention.* http://www.thecommunityguide.org/obesity/index.html (accessed June 8, 2009).

CDC. 2006b. *Guide to Community Preventive Services: Promoting Physical Activity.* http://www.thecommunityguide.org/pa/index.html (accessed June 8, 2009).

Cleland, V. J., A. Timperio, and D. Crawford. 2008. Are perceptions of the physical and social environment associated with mothers' walking for leisure and for transport? A longitudinal study. *Preventive Medicine* 47(2):188–193.

Davison, K. K., and C. T. Lawson. 2006. Do attributes in the physical environment influence children's physical activity? A review of the literature. *International Journal of Behavioral Nutrition and Physical Activity* 3.

Davison, K. K., J. L. Werder, and C. T. Lawson. 2008. Children's active commuting to school: Current knowledge and future directions. *Preventing Chronic Disease* 5(3):A100.

Day, K. 2006. Active living and social justice: Planning for physical activity in low-income, black, and Latino communities. *Journal of the American Planning Association* 72(1):88–99.

Donnelly, J. E., J. L. Greene, C. A. Gibson, B. K. Smith, R. A. Washburn, D. K. Sullivan, et al. 2009. Physical activity across the curriculum (PAAC): a randomized controlled trial to promote physical activity and diminish overweight and obesity in elementary school children. *Preventive Medicine* 49(2):336–341.

Dudas, R. A., and M. Crocetti. 2008. Association of bicycling and childhood overweight status. *Ambulatory Pediatrics* 8(6):392–395.

Elkins, W. L., D. A. Cohen, L. M. Koralewicz, and S. N. Taylor. 2004. After school activities, overweight, and obesity among inner city youth. *Journal of Adolescence* 27(2):181–189.

Ferreira, I., K. Van Der Horst, W. Wendel-Vos, S. Kremers, F. J. Van Lenthe, and J. Brug. 2007. Environmental correlates of physical activity in youth—a review and update. *Obesity Reviews* 8(2):129–154.

Floriani, V., and C. Kennedy. 2008. Promotion of physical activity in children. *Current Opinion in Pediatrics* 20(1):90–95.

Frank, L. D., M. A. Andresen, and T. L. Schmid. 2004. Obesity relationships with community design, physical activity, and time spent in cars. *American Journal of Preventive Medicine* 27(2):87–96.

Goran, M. I., and M. S. Treuth. 2001. Energy expenditure, physical activity, and obesity in children. *Pediatric Clinics of North America* 48(4):931–953.

Gordon-Larsen, P., R. G. McMurray, and B. M. Popkin. 2000. Determinants of adolescent physical activity and inactivity patterns. *Pediatrics* 105(6):E83.

Gordon-Larsen, P., M. C. Nelson, P. Page, and B. M. Popkin. 2006. Inequality in the built environment underlies key health disparities in physical activity and obesity. *Pediatrics* 117(2):417–424.

Grow, H. M., B. E. Saelens, J. Kerr, N. H. Durant, G. J. Norman, and J. F. Sallis. 2008. Where are youth active? Roles of proximity, active transport, and built environment. *Medicine and Science in Sports and Exercise* 40(12):2071–2079.

Handy, S. 2005. Smart growth and the transportation–land use connection: What does the research tell us? *International Regional Science Review* 28(2):146–167.

Handy, S., and K. Clifton. 2007. Planning and the built environment: Implications for obesity prevention. In *Handbook of obesity prevention: A resource for health professionals*. New York: Springer Publishing.

Handy, S., and G. Tal. 2008. Children's biking for non-school purposes: Getting to soccer games in Davis, CA. *Transportation Research Record* 2074:40–45.

HHS and USDA (U.S. Department of Health and Human Services and U.S. Department of Agriculture). 2008. *Physical Activity Guidelines for Americans*. http://www.health.gov/paguidelines/guidelines/default.aspx (accessed May 19, 2009).

Hoefer, W. R., T. L. McKenzie, J. F. Sallis, S. J. Marshall, and T. L. Conway. 2001. Parental provision of transportation for adolescent physical activity. *American Journal of Preventive Medicine* 21(1):48–51.

IOM (Institute of Medicine). 2005. *Preventing Childhood Obesity: Health in the Balance*. Washington, DC: The National Academies Press.

IOM. 2006. *Food Marketing to Children and Youth: Threat or Opportunity?* Washington, DC: The National Academies Press.

Jackson, D. M., K. Djafarian, J. Stewart, and J. R. Speakman 2009. Increased television viewing is associated with elevated body fatness but not with lower total energy expenditure in children. *American Journal of Clinical Nutrition* 89:1031–1036.

Kaczynskl, A. T., and K. A. Henderson. 2008. Parks and recreation settings and active living: A review of associations with physical activity function and intensity. *Journal of Physical Activity and Health* 5(4):619–632.

Kerr, J., D. Rosenberg, J. F. Sallis, B. E. Saelens, L. D. Frank, and T. L. Conway. 2006. Active commuting to school: Associations with environment and parental concerns. *Medicine and Science in Sports and Exercise* 38(4):787–794.

Lara, A., A. K. Yancey, R. Tapia-Conye, Y. Flores, P. Kuri-Morales, R. Mistry, E. Subirats, and W. J. McCarthy. 2008. Pausa para tu salud: Reduction of weight and waistlines by integrating exercise breaks into workplace organizational routine. *Preventing Chronic Disease* 5(1):A12.

Laurson, K. R., J. C. Eisenmann, G. J. Welk, E. E. Wickel, D. A. Gentile, and D. A. Walsh. 2008. Combined influence of physical activity and screen time recommendations on childhood overweight. *Journal of Pediatrics* 153(2):209–214.

Lee, C., and A. V. Moudon. 2008. Neighbourhood design and physical activity. *Building Research and Information* 36(5):395–411.

Lee, I. M., and D. M. Buchner. 2008. The importance of walking to public health. *Medicine and Science in Sports and Exercise* 40(Suppl. 7):S512–S518.

McDonald, N. C. 2007. Active transportation to school. Trends among U.S. Schoolchildren, 1969–2001. *American Journal of Preventive Medicine* 32(6):509–516.

Mota, J., M. Almeida, P. Santos, and J. C. Ribeiro. 2005. Perceived neighborhood environments and physical activity in adolescents. *Preventive Medicine* 41(5–6):834–836.

Must, A., and D. J. Tybor. 2005. Physical activity and sedentary behavior: A review of longitudinal studies of weight and adiposity in youth. *International Journal of Obesity* 29(Suppl. 2):S84–S96.

Powell, L. M., S. Slater, F. J. Chaloupka, and D. Harper. 2006. Availability of physical activity-related facilities and neighborhood demographic and socioeconomic characteristics: A national study. *American Journal of Public Health* 96(9):1676–1680.

Roberts, D. F., U. G. Foehr, and V. Rideout. 2005. *Generation M: Media in the Lives of 8–18 year olds*. http://www.kff.org/entmedia/7251.cfm (accessed June 8, 2009).

Saelens, B. E., and S. L. Handy. 2008. Built environment correlates of walking: A review. *Medicine and Science in Sports and Exercise* 40(Suppl. 7):S550–S566.

Saelens, B. E., J. F. Sallis, J. B. Black, and D. Chen. 2003. Neighborhood-based differences in physical activity: An environment scale evaluation. *American Journal of Public Health* 93(9):1552–1558.

Sallis, J., and K. Glanz. 2009. Physical activity and food environments: Solutions to the obesity epidemic. *The Milbank Quarterly* 87(1):123–154.

Sallis, J. F., J. J. Prochaska, and W. C. Taylor. 2000. A review of correlates of physical activity of children and adolescents. *Medicine and Science in Sports and Exercise* 32(5):963–975.

Seefeldt, V., R. M. Malina, and M. A. Clark. 2002. Factors affecting levels of physical activity in adults. *Sports Medicine* 32(3):143–168.

Weintraub, D. L., E. C. Tirumalai, K. F. Haydel, M. Fujimoto, J. E. Fulton, and T. N. Robinson. 2008. Team sports for overweight children: The Stanford sports to prevent obesity randomized trial (sport). *Archives of Pediatrics and Adolescent Medicine* 162(3):232–237.

Weir, L. A., D. Etelson, and D. A. Brand. 2006. Parents' perceptions of neighborhood safety and children's physical activity. *Preventive Medicine* 43(3):212–217.

Yancey, A. 2007. Social ecological influences on obesity control: Instigating problems and informing potential solutions. *Obesity Management* 3(2):74–79.

Zheng, Y. 2008. The benefit of public transportation: Physical activity to reduce obesity and ecological footprint. *Preventive Medicine* 46(1):4–5.

A

Glossary

As of Right: Zoning standards that are determined in advance of development and are self-enforcing. These types of development do not require special approval from a government agency.

Body Mass Index (BMI): One of the most commonly used measures for defining overweight and obesity, calculated as weight in kilograms divided by height in meters squared.

Built Environment: Encompasses all of the man-made elements of the physical environment, including buildings, infrastructure, and other physical elements created or modified by people and the functional use, arrangement in space, and aesthetic qualities of these elements.

Calorie-Dense, Nutrient-Poor Foods: Foods and beverages that contribute few vitamins and minerals to the diet, but contain substantial amounts of fat and/or sugar and are high in calories. Consumption of these foods, such as sugar-sweetened beverages, candy, and chips, may contribute to excess calorie intake and unwanted weight gain in children.

Complete Streets: Streets that support all users—motorists, bicyclists, pedestrians, transit users, young, old, and disabled—by featuring sidewalks, bicycle lanes, wide shoulders, crosswalks, and other features. Complete streets enable safe, attractive, and comfortable access and travel.

Conditional Use Permit: A variance granted to a property owner that allows a use otherwise prevented by zoning, through a public hearing process. These permits allow a city or county to consider special uses of land that may be essential or desirable to a particular community but are not allowed as a matter of right within a zoning district. These permits can also control certain uses that could have detrimental effects on a community or neighboring properties. They provide flexibility within a zoning ordinance.

Connectivity: The directness of travel to destinations. Sidewalks and paths that are in good condition and without gaps can promote connectivity.

Density: Population per unit of area measure.

Dietary Guidelines for Americans: The Dietary Guidelines for Americans have been published jointly every 5 years since 1980 by the Department of Health and Human Services (HHS) and the Department of Agriculture (USDA). The Guidelines provide authoritative advice for people 2 years and older on how good dietary habits can promote health and reduce risk for major chronic diseases. They serve as the basis for federal nutrition assistance and nutrition education programs.

Discretionary Calories: The number of calories in one's "energy allowance" after one consumes sufficient amounts of foods and beverages to meet one's daily calorie and nutrient needs while promoting weight maintenance.

Energy-Dense Foods: Foods that are high in calories.

Exactions: Requirements placed on developers as a condition of development approval, generally falling into two categories: impact fees (see below) or physical exactions such as dedication of land or provision of infrastructure. Exactions must be related to the expected impacts of a project. For example, new homes create the need for more parks and schools, and an exaction might dedicate land in the developer's plans for more parks and schools.

Food Access: The extent to which a community can supply people with the food needed for health. Communities with poor food access lack the resources necessary to supply people with the food needed for a healthy lifestyle. Availability of high-quality, affordable food and close proximity to food stores increase food access.

Form-Based Code: A method of regulating development to achieve a specific urban form. Form-based codes create a predictable public realm primarily by controlling physical form, with a lesser focus on land use, through city or county regulations.

Health Disparities/Inequities: Terms used to describe differences in quality of health and health care across racial, ethnic, and socioeconomic groups.

Healthy Eating Environment: An environment that provides access to and encourages the consumption of healthy foods, as described by the Dietary Guidelines for Americans.

Healthy Equity: The fair distribution of health determinants, outcomes, and resources within and among segments of the population, regardless of social standing.

Home Zone: A residential street or group of streets that is designed to operate primarily as a space for social use. The needs of residents take priority over the needs of car drivers. Home zones are designed to be shared by pedestrians, playing children, bicyclists, and low-speed motor vehicles. Traffic-calming methods such as speed humps are avoided in favor of methods that make slower speeds more natural to drivers, rather than an imposition. Home zones encourage children's play and neighborhood interaction and also increase road safety.

Impact Fee: A monetary exaction placed on developers related to the expected impacts of a project. For example, to lessen the effect of increased traffic at a new shopping center, a developer might be required to pay an impact fee that would be used for construction of a left-turn lane and traffic lights.

Macronutrients: Nutrients needed in relatively large quantities, such as protein, carbohydrates, and fat.

Micronutrients: Nutrients needed in relatively small quantities, such as vitamins and minerals.

Mixed Land Use: A mixed land use development incorporates many sectors of a community, including retail, office, and residential. Communities with a balanced mix of land use give residents the option to walk, bike, or take transit to nearby attractions.

Nutrient-Dense Foods: Foods that provide substantial amounts of vitamins, minerals, and other health-promoting components such as fiber and relatively few calories. Foods that are low in nutrient density supply calories but no or small amounts of vitamins, minerals, and health-promoting components.

Obesity and Overweight: Children and adolescents are defined as obese if they have a body mass index (BMI) equal to or greater than the 95th percentile for their age and sex, and overweight if they have a BMI at the 85th percentile to less than the 95th percentile for their age and sex, according to growth charts (http://www.cdc.gov/growthcharts).

Physical Activity: Body movement produced by the contraction of muscle that increases energy expenditure above the resting level.

Pocket Park: A small park frequently created on a vacant building lot or on a small, irregular piece of land, sometimes created as a component of the public space requirement of large building projects. Pocket parks provide greenery, a place to sit outdoors, and sometimes playground equipment. They may be created around a monument, historic marker, or art project.

Retrofit: Modification of infrastructure and facilities in existing areas of the community rather than the provision of infrastructure and facilities in new areas of development.

Road Diet: Involves reducing the amount of lanes in a road to include a bike lane and/or sidewalks. Road diets are intended to slow traffic and make the road safer for pedestrians and cyclists.

Smart Growth: An approach to urban planning that is more town centered and transit and pedestrian oriented, and has a greater mix of housing, commercial, and retail uses. It also preserves open space and many other environmental amenities.

Social Environment: Includes interactions with family, friends, coworkers, and others in the community. It also encompasses social institutions, such as the workplace, places of worship, and schools. Housing, public transportation, law enforcement, and the presence or absence of violence in the community are among other components of the social environment. The social environment has a profound effect on individual health, as well as on the health of the larger community, and is unique because of cultural customs; language; and personal, religious, or spiritual beliefs. At the same time, individuals and their behaviors contribute to the quality of the social environment (definition from *Healthy People 2010*).

Social Marketing: Using the same marketing principles that are used to sell products to consumers to "sell" ideas, attitudes, and behaviors. Social marketing is often used to change health behaviors.

Stranger Danger: The perceived danger to children presented by strangers. The phrase is intended to sum up the various concerns associated with the threat presented by unknown adults.

Traffic Calming: Measures that attempt to slow traffic speeds and increase pedestrian and bicycle traffic through physical devices designed to be self-enforcing. These include speed humps and bumps, raised intersections, road narrowing, bends and deviations in a road, medians, central islands, and traffic circles.

VERB Campaign: A national, multicultural, social marketing campaign to increase and maintain physical activity among tweens. It was coordinated by the U.S. Department of Health and Human Services and and the Centers for Disease Control and Prevention and ran from 2002 to 2006.

B

Toolkits and Related Resources

Aboelata, M., L. Mikkelsen, L. Cohen, S. Fernandes, M. Silver, L. Parks, J. DuLong. 2004. *The Built Environment and Health—11 Profiles of Neighborhood Transformation.* http://www.preventioninstitute.org/pdf/BE_full_document_110304.pdf (accessed May 27, 2009).

ASTHO (Association of State and Territorial Health Officials). 2006. *State Options for Reducing Overweight and Obesity.* Washington, DC: ASTHO.

CDC (Centers for Disease Control and Prevention). 2006. *Guide to Community Preventive Services.* www.thecommunityguide.org (accessed June 10, 2009).

The Finance Project. 2004. *Financing Childhood Obesity Prevention Programs: Federal Funding Sources and other Strategies.* http://www.financeproject.org/Publications/obesityprevention.pdf (accessed August 4, 2009).

Harvard Pilgrim Health Care Foundation. 2008. *Tipping the Scales in Favor of our Children.* https://www.harvardpilgrim.org/pls/portal/docs/PAGE/MEMBERS/FOUNDATION/GROWING_UP_HEALTHY/TIPPINGSCALES/TIPPING_SCALES.PDF (accessed May 27, 2009).

Healthy Eating by Design. 2008. *Lessons from the Field: Promoting Healthy Eating in Communities.* http://www.activelivingbydesign.org/sites/default/files/HEbD_Lessons_from_communities_FINAL2.pdf (accessed May 27, 2009).

Heroux, J. 2005. *Lessons Learned: Promoting Physical Activity at the Community Level.* http://www.rwjf.org/files/publications/LessonsLearned_PhysicalActivity_GRR.pdf (accessed May 28, 2009).

HHS (U.S. Department of Health and Human Services). 2006. *Promoting Physical Activity and Healthy Nutrition in Afterschool Settings: Strategies for Program Leaders and Policy Makers.* http://nccic.acf.hhs.gov/afterschool/fitness_nutrition.pdf (accessed May 27, 2009).

ICMA (International City/County Management Association). 2006. *Community Health and Food Access: The Local Government Role.* http://www.icma.org/upload/library/2006-09/%7B5CD4101C-2803-4655-9A51-465461B3C897%7D.pdf (accessed May 27, 2009).

Leadership for Healthy Communities. 2007. *Improving Access to Healthy Foods: A Guide for Policy-makers.* http://www.rwjf.org/files/research/accesshealthyfoodslhc2007.pdf (accessed May 27, 2009).

Leadership for Healthy Communities. 2007. *Increasing Active Living: A Guide for Policy-makers.* http://www.rwjf.org/files/research/activelivinglhc2007.pdf (accessed May 27, 2009).

Local Government Commission. *Cultivating Community Gardens: The Role of Local Government in Creating Healthy, Livable Neighborhoods.* http://www.lgc.org/freepub/docs/community_design/fact_sheets/community_gardens.pdf (accessed May 27, 2009).

Local Government Commission and the Cities, Counties and School Partnership. 2007. *Healthy Kids, Healthy Communities: School and Local Government Collaborations.* http://www.lgc.org/freepub/docs/community_design/fact_sheets/Healthy_Kids_Healthy_Communities.pdf (accessed May 27, 2009).

NACo (National Association of Counties). 2005. *County Government Approaches to Combating Youth Obesity, Encouraging Physical Activity, and Creating Healthy Communities.* http://www.naco.org/Content/ContentGroups/Programs_and_Projects/Community_Development/Center_for_Sustainable_Communities/Final_Youth_Obesity_SurveyReport.pdf (accessed May 27, 2009).

NACo. 2008. *Transportation Solutions to Create Active, Healthy Counties: Collaboration for Childhood Obesity Prevention.* http://www.naco.org/Template.cfm?Section=New_Technical_Assistance&template=/ContentManagement/ContentDisplay.cfm&ContentID=27724 (accessed May 27, 2009).

NALBOH (National Association of Local Boards of Health). 2006. *Land Use Planning for Public Health: The Role of Local Boards of Health in Community Design and Development.* http://www.activeliving.org/files/NALBOH_land_use_report.pdf (accessed May 28, 2009).

NALEO (National Association of Latino Elected Officials). *Obesity in your Community.* http://www.naleo.org/downloads/HealthToolKit.pdf (accessed May 27, 2009).

New Orleans Food Policy Advisory Committee. 2007. *Building Healthy Communities: Expanding Access to Fresh Food Retail.* http://www.sph.tulane.edu/PRC/Files/FPAC%20Report%20Final.pdf (accessed May 27, 2009).

NLC (National League of Cities). 2006. Combating childhood obesity, Issue #8. *Action Kit for Municipal Leaders.* http://www.nlc.org/ASSETS/FC9AD61015584D1789198583E6C888E8/IYEF_Action_Kit_Childhood_Obesity.pdf (accessed May 27, 2009).

PolicyLink and Local Initiatives Support Corporation. 2007. *Grocery Store Attraction Strategies: A Resource Guide for Community Activists and Local Governments*. http://www.lisc.org/bay_area/assets/grocerymanual_10408.pdf (accessed May 28, 2009).

Prevention Institute. *ENACT (Environmental Nutrition and Activity Community Tool)*. http://www.preventioninstitute.org/sa/enact/members/index.php (accessed May 27, 2009).

Prevention Institute. 2008. *Promising Strategies for Creating Healthy Eating and Active Living Environments*. http://www.preventioninstitute.org/documents/promisingstrategies.pdf (accessed May 28, 2009).

Public Health Law and Policy. 2008. *How to Create and Implement Healthy General Plans—a Toolkit for Building Healthy, Vibrant Communities through Land Use Policy Change*. http://www.healthyplanning.org/healthygp_toolkit/HealthyGP_TOC.pdf (accessed September 10, 2009).

RE-AIM. www.re-aim.org (accessed June 10, 2009).

Rosenthal, J. 2005. *Enhancing State and Local Capacity to Promote Healthy Weight in Children: Addressing Disparities in the Real World*. http://www.nashp.org/Files/GNL60_obesity_disparities_final_6.7.05.pdf (accessed May 28, 2009).

Rosenthal, J., and D. Chang. 2004. *State Approaches to Childhood Obesity: A Snapshot of Promising Practices and Lessons Learned*. http://www.nashp.org/Files/Obesity_final_with_correct_appendix_C.pdf (accessed May 28, 2009).

RWJF (Robert Wood Johnson Foundation). 2007. *Balance—a Report on State Action to Promote Nutrition, Increase Physical Activity and Prevent Obesity*. http://www.rwjf.org/childhoodobesity/product.jsp?id=31471 (accessed May 27, 2009).

Swinburn, B., T. Gill, and S. Kumanyika. 2005. Obesity prevention: A proposed framework for translating evidence into action. *Obesity Reviews* 6(1):23–33.

Texas Department of State Health Services. 2006. *Texas Obesity Policy Portfolio*. http://www.dshs.state.tx.us/cpcpi/pdf/obesityportfolio.pdf (accessed May 28, 2009).

Trust for America's Health. 2008. *F as in Fat: How Obesity Policies are Failing in America*. http://healthyamericans.org/reports/obesity2008/Obesity2008Report.pdf (accessed May 27, 2009).

The United States Conference of Mayors. 2008. *Mayors' Guide to Fighting Childhood Obesity*. http://usmayors.org/chhs/healthycities/documents/guide-20080326.pdf (accessed May 27, 2009).

Zenzola, T. 2005. *Land Use Planning and Community Design: The Role of Local Public Health Agencies. A Focus Group Report*. National Association of County and City Health Officials. http://www.naccho.org/topics/environmental/landuseplanning/upload/land-use-planning-and-local-public-health-officials.pdf (accessed November 17, 2009).

C

Methodology

The committee was convened to develop a set of recommended childhood obesity prevention practices for local governments. In tackling the committee's charge, a set of over 600 articles from peer-reviewed published literature and reports from organizations relevant to local governments was identified. The focus of the literature review was to identify potential childhood obesity prevention actions for consideration by the committee, retrieve review articles and seminal articles on the evidence available on potential actions, and find criteria and tools that would be useful in making determinations on the most promising actions.

Scopus and the Transportation Research Information Services (TRIS) online database were primarily used to search the literature, supplemented by EMBASE, PsycINFO, and Medline. **Scopus** is a multidisciplinary research tool indexing more than 15,000 peer-reviewed journals from 4,000 publishers. Subject areas covered by Scopus include chemistry, physics, mathematics, engineering, life and health sciences, social sciences, psychology, economics, biological, agricultural and environmental sciences, and general sciences. The **TRIS** database is the world's largest and most comprehensive bibliographic resource on transportation information. TRIS is produced and maintained by the Transportation Research Board at the National Academy of Sciences. **EMBASE** (Excerpta Medica) is a major biomedical and pharmaceutical database containing more than 9 million records from over 4,000 journals. This database indexes international journals in the following fields: drug research, pharmacology, pharmaceutics, toxicology, clinical and experimental human medicine, health policy and management, public health, occupational health, environmental health, drug dependence and abuse, psychiatry, forensic medicine, and biomedical engineering/instrumentation. **PsycINFO** is a database of psychological literature and it contains more than 1,900,000 records including citations and summaries of journal articles, book chapters, books, and technical reports, as well as citations to dissertations, all in the field of psychology and psychological aspects of related disciplines. **Medline** is the U.S. National Library of Medicine's bibliographic database, covering the fields of medicine, nursing, dentistry, veterinary medicine, the health care system, and the preclinical sciences. PubMed, provides online access to over 12 million Medline citations. Medline contains bibliographic citations and author abstracts from more than 4,600 biomedical journals published in the United States and 70 other countries.

The initial search strategy paired the terms obesity and overweight with terms related to food access (neighborhoods, supermarkets, grocery stores, farmers' markets, breastfeeding, menu labeling, after-school programs, youth programs, community gardens, federal food programs), and terms related to physical activity, including topics concerning the built environment (recreation, parks, playgrounds, planning, sprawl, zoning, walkability, paths, trails) and transportation (sidewalks, roads, traffic patterns, safety, complete streets).

A scan also was conducted to identify recommended childhood obesity prevention actions that have been undertaken in the last ten years by organizations that work with local governments. These organizations included the National Association of County and City Health Officials (NACCHO), Centers for Disease Control and Prevention (CDC), Leadership for Healthy Communities, International City/County Management Association (ICMA), National League of Cities, National Association of Counties (NACo), Local Government Commission, Association of State and Territorial Health Officials (ASTHO), Prevention Institute, U.S Conference of Mayors, and National Association of Latino Elected Officials (NALEO). These organizations have all published reports and/or toolkits that discuss what local governments can do to prevent childhood obesity. The committee also reviewed several sets of criteria and tools developed by others that could be relevant to the committee's task of making determinations on the most promising actions. (A list of these resources can be found in Appendix B.)

In addition, the committee invited presentations from experts on the role of local government in childhood obesity prevention (see Appendix F).

Based on these searches and presentations, a broad spectrum of action steps and the research on them was compiled. These actions clustered around 15 distinct strategies.

Informed by these efforts, the committee developed criteria for consideration as it reviewed specific strategies and action steps for whether they had the potential to make a positive difference in healthy eating or physical activity. The committee's criteria were that the strategies and actions must be

- Within the jurisdiction of local governments;
- Likely to affect children directly;
- Targeted to changing the food or physical activity environments of children outside the school walls and the school day (in accordance with the committee's charge);
- Actionable based on the experience of local governments or knowledgeable sources that work with local governments; and
- Likely to make positive contributions to the achievement of healthy eating and/or optimum physical activity based on research evidence or, where such evidence is lacking or limited, have a logical connection with the achievement of healthier eating or increased physical activity.

Using the available evidence, the committee took into account the following characteristics of the strategies and actions: their evidence of effectiveness and effect size; outcomes and externalities; potential reach, impact, and cost; and feasibility. The committee made a final assessment and determination of its recommended actions (58 in all) using a nominal voting procedure. Lastly, the committee chose 12 action steps it believes have the most promising potential to make a difference, based on consideration of the criteria described above and the results of the nominal voting.

D

Assessing the Evidence for Childhood Obesity Prevention Action Steps

The purpose of this appendix is to help the reader understand the nature of the evidence for the action steps.

To determine the most promising childhood obesity prevention actions for local governments, the committee reviewed numerous research articles from peer-reviewed published literature as well as reports from organizations that work with local governments on childhood obesity prevention. In order to be recommended, action steps were selected that local governments generally have the authority to carry out. In addition, they had to have a direct impact on children and they had to be actions that had been implemented by local governments or had been recommended by knowledgeable sources as actions for local governments. Finally, the recommended actions had to be ones that were likely to make positive contributions to the achievement of healthy eating and/or optimal physical activity based on research evidence or, where that was lacking or limited, have a logical connection with the achievement of healthier eating or increased physical activity.

The committee considered three categories of evidence, realizing that some actions had multiple types of evidence:

- Intervention evidence: A few of the actions have been tested in randomized intervention studies. Randomized controlled trials are not feasible for many community efforts and while recognizing the value of this type of research, the committee also realized the practical constraints that make it infeasible to examine the effectiveness of all types of actions in this way.

- Observational evidence: A number of the action steps have been discussed in published studies that provide observations on how an action fared in one community or population, or examine associations of community characteristics with healthy eating, physical activity, or weight in a particular community or set of communities.

- Limited evidence: Some action steps do not have direct research evidence. The selection of those actions was based on related evidence indicating that they are likely to have a positive effect on healthy eating and/or optimal physical activity. An example would be the action step to "create incentive programs to attract supermarkets and grocery stores to underserved neighborhoods." Although there is no direct research evidence on the impact of incentive programs to attract supermarkets and grocery stores to these neighborhoods, there is observational evidence (cited in the rationale for Strategy 1: Retail Outlets) that neighborhood residents who have better access to supermarkets tend to have healthier diets and lower levels of obesity.

The 15 strategies recommended in the report are listed below, with a characterization under each one of the type of evidence supporting the action steps for that strategy. In addition, particular attention is paid to the types of evidence supporting each of the 12 action steps that the committee highlighted.

Actions For Healthy Eating

GOAL 1: IMPROVE ACCESS TO AND CONSUMPTION OF HEALTHY, SAFE, AND AFFORDABLE FOODS

Strategy 1: Increase community access to healthy foods through supermarkets, grocery stores, and convenience/corner stores.

All of the action steps under this strategy have limited evidence. However, the action step to "create incentive programs to attract supermarkets and grocery stores to underserved neighborhoods" was highlighted by the committee as one of its 12 action steps for special consideration. As mentioned in the above example, there is observational evidence that neighborhood residents who have better access to supermarkets tend to have healthier diets and lower levels of obesity. This highlighted action step is likely to make positive contributions to the achievement of healthier eating. It has the potential to reach a large population and several cities are in the process of implementing incentive programs. There is growing interest in the implementation of this action and increased research in this area would be useful.

Strategy 2: Improve the availability and identification of healthful foods in restaurants.

There is observational evidence supporting the action steps related to menu labeling. The committee's highlighted action step under this strategy: "Require menu labeling in chain restaurants to provide consumers with calorie information on in-store menus and menu boards" is supported by observational evidence that calorie information may have a positive influence on food choices in a restaurant setting. This action step has the potential to reach a large segment of the population and is being implemented by a number of restaurant chains. There is a growing interest in the implementation of this action and increased research in this area would be very useful. On the other hand, there is limited evidence for the action step on offering incentives to restaurants that promote healthier options.

Strategy 3: Promote efforts to provide fruits and vegetables in a variety of settings, such as farmers' markets, farm stands, mobile markets, community gardens, and youth-focused gardens.

There is intervention and/or observational evidence for all of the action steps under this strategy except one: "Develop community-based activities that link procurement of affordable healthy food with improving skills in purchasing and preparing food." As with all of the steps with limited evidence, this categorization is a reflection of the lack of published research.

Strategy 4: Ensure that publicly run entities such as after-school programs, child care facilities, recreation centers, and local government worksites implement policies and practices to promote healthy foods and beverages and reduce or eliminate the availability of calorie-dense, nutrient-poor foods.

For this strategy, the action steps listed have limited evidence. The committee highlighted one action step under this strategy: "Mandate and implement strong nutrition standards for foods and beverages available in government-run or regulated after-school programs, recreation centers, parks, and child care facilities" because of the potential reach of such standard-setting and the feasibility of doing so in government-run and or regulated programs. There is growing interest in the implementation of such an action, and more research on the effectiveness of nutrition standards in these settings would be helpful.

Strategy 5: Increase participation in federal, state, and local government nutrition assistance programs (e.g., WIC, school breakfast and lunch, the Child and Adult Care Food Program [CACFP], the Afterschool Snacks Program, the Summer Food Service Program, SNAP).

There is limited evidence on the action steps under this strategy. However, several observational studies show associations between nutrition program participation and lower BMI.

Strategy 6: Encourage breastfeeding and promote breastfeeding-friendly communities.

The majority of the action steps under this strategy have limited evidence. However, there is observational evidence supporting the action step: "Adopt practices in city and county hospitals that are consistent with the Baby-Friendly Hospital Initiative."

Strategy 7: Increase access to free, safe drinking water in public places to encourage water consumption in place of sugar-sweetened beverages.

A recent study provides intervention evidence that supports the action steps under this strategy. The committee highlighted the action step: "Adopt building codes to require access to, and maintenance of, fresh drinking water fountains." The research showed an increase in water consumption and a reduction in risk of overweight in school children with the installation of water fountains in their building. Building code changes have a broad reach. There is strong interest in increasing water consumption as an obesity prevention strategy, and more research in this area would be helpful.

GOAL 2: REDUCE ACCESS TO AND CONSUMPTION OF CALORIE-DENSE, NUTRIENT-POOR FOODS

Strategy 8: Implement fiscal policies and local ordinances to discourage the consumption of calorie-dense, nutrient-poor foods and beverages (e.g., taxes, incentives, land use and zoning regulations).

Overall, the action steps listed for this strategy have limited evidence. However, there is some observational evidence supporting the use of land use and zoning policies related to fast food establishments near schools and residential areas. The committee highlighted the action step: "Implement a tax strategy to discourage consumption of foods and beverages that have minimal nutritional value, such as sugar-sweetened beverages." Although there is limited evidence on the impact of this action step, there is growing interest in its potential to reduce obesity, and its reach is likely to be broad. More research related to the implementation of this action step would be useful.

GOAL 3: RAISE AWARENESS ABOUT THE IMPORTANCE OF HEALTHY EATING TO PREVENT CHILDHOOD OBESITY

Strategy 9: Promote media and social marketing campaigns on healthy eating and childhood obesity prevention.

There is intervention evidence supporting the action step that the committee highlighted for special consideration under this strategy: "Develop media campaigns, utilizing multiple channels to promote healthy eating using consistent messages." In addition, this action step has the potential to reach a broad population, and more research on its impact would be valuable. The rest of the action steps under this strategy have limited evidence.

Actions for Increasing Physical Activity

GOAL 1: ENCOURAGE PHYSICAL ACTIVITY

Strategy 1: Encourage walking and bicycling for transportation and recreation through improvements in the built environment.

Most of the action steps under this strategy are supported by observational evidence, including the action step the committee highlighted under this strategy: "Plan, build, and maintain a network of sidewalks and street crossings that creates a safe and comfortable walking environment and that connects to schools, parks, and other destinations." Besides being supported by published research evidence, including recommendations by CDC's Task Force on Community Preventive Services, this action step has the potential for reaching a large segment of the population.

Strategy 2: Promote programs that support walking and bicycling for transportation.

The majority of action steps under this strategy are supported by observational evidence. There is limited evidence on the impact of improved access to bicycles and related equipment or increased transit use through reduced fares for children on physical activity. There are two action steps under this strategy that were highlighted by the committee: "Adopt community policing strategies that improve safety and security of streets, especially in higher crime neighborhoods" and "Collaborate with schools to develop and implement a *Safe Routes to School* program to increase the number of children safely walking and bicycling to schools." Both are supported by observational evidence, and both have the potential to reach large numbers of people. More research in these areas would be helpful.

Strategy 3: Promote other forms of recreational physical activity.

The action steps under this strategy are supported by observational and intervention evidence. Two of the committee-highlighted action steps: "Build and maintain parks and playgrounds that are safe and attractive for playing, and in close proximity to residential areas" and "Adopt community policing strategies that improve safety and security for park use, especially in higher crime neighborhoods" are supported by observational evidence. The other highlighted strategy: "Collaborate with school districts and other organizations to establish joint use of facilities agreements for allowing playing fields, playgrounds and recreation centers to be used by community residents when schools are closed" is supported in part by intervention evidence from a study that examined the impact of opening neighborhood schoolyards on weekends and after school for children's use. All three action steps have the potential for broad reach in the community, are of great interest to communities, and research on their effectiveness would be very useful.

Strategy 4: Promote policies that build physical activity into daily routines.

Overall, there is limited evidence for the action steps under this strategy, although there is observational evidence supporting the action step: "Develop worksite policies and practices that build physical activity into routines." The committee highlighted for special consideration the action step: "Institute regulatory policies mandating minimum play space, physical equipment, and duration of play in preschool, after-school, and child-care programs." This action step has limited evidence but there is observational evidence that the availability of play equipment increases physical activity in child care centers. This action step has the potential for broad reach because of the large number of children being cared for outside the home, and research on the effectiveness of this action step would be very useful. There is also a growing interest in influencing children's physical activity in child care centers and after school programs.

GOAL 2: DECREASE SEDENTARY BEHAVIOR

Strategy 5: Promote policies that reduce sedentary screen time.

There is observational evidence supporting the action step under this strategy. Moreover, the CDC's Task Force on Community Preventive Services recommends behavioral interventions to reduce screen time.

GOAL 3: RAISE AWARENESS OF THE IMPORTANCE OF INCREASING PHYSICAL ACTIVITY

Strategy 6: Develop a social marketing program that emphasizes the multiple benefits for children and families of sustained physical activity.

The action step for this strategy that recommends "a social marketing program that emphasizes the multiple benefits for children and families of sustained physical activity" is supported by intervention evidence. The other action steps under this strategy have limited evidence.

As mentioned often in this report, the evidence base for local government actions is limited in certain areas, but steadily accumulating. The shortcomings in the evidence base should not discourage action, but should encourage continuing research, evaluation, and analysis whenever possible, especially in those areas in which evidence is lacking. When local governments evaluate the results of their childhood obesity prevention actions, it is important to ensure that this information is broadly disseminated.

E

Statement of Task

An ad hoc committee of the Institute of Medicine will examine evidence on childhood obesity prevention efforts by local government entities, with a focus on identifying promising practices, and will develop a set of recommended practices for disseminating to local governments broadly. The audience includes mayors; county, city, or township commissioners or other officials; local health departments; local boards of health; city and transportation planners; and other relevant local commissions and public entities. This study will draw from and build on relevant Institute of Medicine (IOM) reports, especially *Preventing Childhood Obesity: Health in the Balance* and *Progress in Preventing Childhood Obesity: How Do We Measure Up?*, as well as secondary sources and seminal primary sources. In carrying out its task the committee will consider the range of childhood obesity prevention efforts that have been considered or implemented by local governments and those that have been evaluated, and from that information will compile a list of promising practices in childhood obesity prevention, noting promising strategies for addressing disparities and disproportionately affected children and youth, identifying other public health benefits, and summarizing successful strategies for sustained funding and financing of obesity prevention initiatives. The committee will develop a succinct report that summarizes the range of local government efforts; identifies and describes rationale for selected promising practices; discusses other relevant public health benefits of these promising practices; and outlines a set of recommendations on priority immediate actions and practices for local governments. As relevant to the task, state government actions may also be considered.

F

Open Session

Committee on Childhood Obesity Prevention Actions for Local Governments

Perspective on Local Government Initiatives
January 27, 2009
3:00–4:45 pm
Irvine, CA

Panel:

- Gerardo Mouet, Executive Director, Parks, Recreation, and Community Services Agency, Santa Ana, CA
- Matthew M. Longjohn, Senior Policy and Political Analyst, CLOCC (Chicago); Adjunct Assistant Professor of Pediatrics, Northwestern University Feinberg School of Medicine; and Institute Fellow and Project Director, Altarum Institute
- Marice Ashe, Director, Public Health Law and Policy, Public Health Institute, Oakland, CA

G

Biographical Sketches

Eduardo J. Sanchez, M.D., M.P.H., FAAFP (*Chair*), is Vice President and Chief Medical Officer for Blue Cross and Blue Shield of Texas. Previously, he was Director of the Institute for Health Policy at the Austin Regional Campus of the School of Public Health in the University of Texas Health Science Center at Houston. He was also previous Commissioner of the Texas Department of State Health Services. Dr. Sanchez received his M.D. from the University of Texas Southwestern Medical School in Dallas and holds an M.P.H. from the University of Texas Health Science Center at Houston School of Public Health and an M.S. in biomedical engineering from Duke University. He holds a B.S. in biomedical engineering and a B.A. in chemistry from Boston University. As Commissioner and Chief Health Officer for the State of Texas, Dr. Sanchez oversaw mental health and substance abuse prevention and treatment programs, disease prevention and bioterrorism preparedness programs, family and community health services programs, and environmental and consumer safety and health-related regulatory programs. Dr. Sanchez is a Fellow of the American Academy of Family Physicians. He practiced clinical medicine in Austin from 1992 to 2001. He also served as Health Authority and Chief Medical Officer for the Austin–Travis County Health and Human Services Department from 1994 to 1998. Dr. Sanchez served on the Institute of Medicine (IOM) Committee on Progress in Preventing Childhood Obesity and is a current member of the IOM Standing Committee on Childhood Obesity Prevention and the IOM Committee on a Comprehensive Review of the DHHS Office of Family Planning Title X Program.

Peggy Beltrone, B.A., is a Cascade County (MT) Commissioner. She is also Chair and Founder of Get Fit Great Falls, an organization that encourages physical activity by organizing free and low-cost outdoor events and providing transportation and equipment for people to get to and use trails. Ms. Beltrone started Get Fit Great Falls in 2004 after attending a U.S. Forest Service recreation summit showcasing a federal effort to use public lands to encourage physical activity. With the forest supervisor at Lewis and Clark National Forest, she began outreach to community members and local health and recreation departments. Those departments and other partners, such as the local hospital, the Girl Scouts, 4-H, and the Great Falls Public School system, have made Get Fit Great Falls a truly collaborative effort. The program has had such success that the U.S. Forest Service held it up as a model in recent congressional testimony. In addition to her work with the program, Ms. Beltrone chaired the National Association of Counties (NACo) Rural Obesity Initiative. A paper addressing the differences involved in approaching childhood obesity in a rural versus an urban setting can be found on the NACo website. Ms. Beltrone is co-chair of NACo's Mobilizing County Officials to Prevent Youth Obesity, an initiative funded by Leadership for Healthy Communities.

Laura K. Brennan, Ph.D., M.P.H., is President and CEO of Transtria, a public health research and consulting company in St. Louis, MO. She is also an assistant professor of Behavioral Science and Health Education in the Department of Community Health at Saint Louis University School of Public Health. Dr. Brennan received her Ph.D. from Saint Louis University. For more than 10 years, she has participated in designing and evaluating community-based initiatives, conducting community-based participatory approaches to intervention and research, developing and communicating health messages, creating and assessing evidence-based intervention strategies, and performing needs assessment through surveys, interviews, and focus groups. She has participated in multiple projects at the national, state, and local levels to facilitate discussions among practitioners (health, transportation, urban planning, parks and recreation, community organizing), researchers, providers, community members and advocacy groups to assist them in planning efforts to address social, economic and environmental influences on health. Dr. Brennan has published 19 peer-reviewed articles studying behaviors and health, she is lead author of *Promoting Healthy Equity: A Resource to Help Communities Address Social Determinants of Health,* and she is a co-author of *Tailoring Health Messages: Customizing Communication with Computer*

Technology. She is active with the Alliance for the Status of Missouri Women, Citizen's for Modern Transit, and the Missouri Family Health Council.

Joseph A. Curtatone, J.D., is serving his third term as mayor of Somerville, Massachusetts. Mr. Curtatone earned his B.A. from Boston College in 1990, and a J.D. from New England School of Law in 1994. Prior to his election as mayor, he had served as an attorney in private practice. As Mayor, he has successfully implemented a wide range of reforms and new programs that have earned Somerville many distinctions from regional and national organizations, including designation by *Boston Globe Magazine* as "the best-run city in Massachusetts" and by America's Promise Alliance as one of the "100 Best Communities for Youth"; the city was also named an All America City in June 2009 by the National Civic League. Under his leadership, Somerville has also earned national recognition for its successful joint effort with Tufts University to implement "Shape Up Somerville," an effective program to reduce the incidence of childhood obesity among the city's elementary school children. The campaign targeted all segments of the community, including schools, city government, civic organizations, community groups, businesses, and other people who live, work, and play in Somerville. His success in Somerville has earned him the presidency of the Massachusetts Mayor's Association, a position on the Board of Directors for the National League of Cities, and as a member of the Metropolitan Mayors Association.

Eric A. Finkelstein, Ph.D., M.H.A., is a health economist for the research organization RTI International in Research Triangle Park, North Carolina. Dr. Finkelstein obtained an M.H.A., and an M.A. and Ph.D. in economics from the University of Washington and a B.A. in mathematics/economics from the University of Michigan, Ann Arbor. His work focuses on the economic causes and consequences of health-related behaviors, with a primary emphasis on obesity. Dr. Finkelstein has published more than 40 peer-reviewed articles on the economics of obesity and related behaviors. His research has been featured on the front page of *USA Today* and has been covered in the *Economist*, the *New York Times*, *Forbes*, the *Washington Post*, and many other newspaper, radio, and television outlets. Dr. Finkelstein also co-wrote the book *The Fattening of America—How the Economy Makes Us Fat, If It Matters, and What to Do About It.* He leads several projects concerning the causes and consequences of obesity and evaluates several obesity prevention programs for the Centers for Disease

Control and Prevention and other agencies. Prior to joining RTI, he was an Agency for Health Care Policy and Research fellow and research scientist with the University of Washington's Department of Family Medicine. He has also taught health economics at Duke University.

Tracy Fox, M.P.H., R.D., is a nutrition and policy consultant and President of Food, Nutrition, and Policy Consultants, LLC. Ms. Fox received her M.P.H. from the University of Pittsburgh Graduate School of Public Health and a B.S. in dietetics from Hood College. Ms. Fox has held positions as Senior Federal Regulatory Manager with the American Dietetic Association, Washington, DC; Food Program Specialist in the Child Nutrition Division and Assistant to the Associate Administrator with the U.S. Department of Agriculture, Food and Nutrition Service, Alexandria, Virginia; Manager of Federal Systems Division with Maximus, Inc., Falls Church, Virginia; Instructor of Food Preparation and Meal Management at Hood College, Frederick, Maryland; and dietitian in food management and clinical dietetics with the U.S. Navy. She is Vice President of the Society for Nutrition Education and serves on the Action for Healthy Kids Partner Steering Committee, is on the board of the Maryland Healthy Schools Coalition, Co-Chaired the Montgomery County School Health Council, and Chaired the Health Committee of the Montgomery County Council of Parent-Teacher Associations. Ms. Fox was a member of the IOM Committee on Nutrition Standards for Foods in School.

Susan L. Handy, Ph.D., is a professor in the Department of Environmental Science and Policy at the University of California at Davis. She is also the director of the Sustainable Transportation Center, part of the federal university transportation centers program. Dr. Handy received a B.S.E. in civil engineering from Princeton University, an M.S. in civil engineering from Stanford University, and her Ph.D. in city and regional planning from the University of California at Berkeley. Her research focuses on the relationships between transportation and land use, particularly the impact of land use on travel behavior, and on strategies for reducing automobile dependence. Her recent work includes a series of studies on bicycling in Davis, examinations of changing policies and practices in regional transportation planning, an exploration of the travel needs of recent immigrants in California, and a study of the effect of cul-de-sacs on children's outdoor play. She currently serves on the National Academies' Committee on Innovations in Travel Demand Modeling and she was a member of the Committee of Telecommunications and Travel Behavior; Committee on Research on Women's Issues in Transportation; Committee for the Prevention of Obesity in Children and Youth; and the Committee on Carbon Monoxide Episodes in Meteorological and Topographical Problem Areas.

James Krieger, M.D., M.P.H., is Chief of the Chronic Disease and Injury Prevention Section at Public Health–Seattle and King County, Clinical Professor of Medicine and Health Services, and Attending Physician at the University of Washington. He received his undergraduate degree at Harvard University, completed medical training at the University of California, San Francisco, and received an M.P.H. from the University of Washington. His recent research work has emphasized interventions to reduce health disparities by addressing social determinants of health. One area of focus is working with public housing and lower-income communities to design and evaluate healthy community interventions that promote physical activity, increase access to healthy foods, and build community. Dr. Krieger has also directed two community chronic disease coalitions which seek to reduce disparities in asthma, diabetes and overweight: Seattle-King County Allies Against Asthma and King County Steps to Health. He is senior leader for the newly funded Kellogg Food and Fitness Initiative that links food systems work with healthy built environments. He directed Seattle Partners for Healthy Communities, a collaboration between community, public health, and the university to conduct community-based participatory research about interventions that address social determinants of health. Dr. Krieger is a nationally recognized expert in housing and health and the development and evaluation of community-based chronic disease control and prevention programs.

Donald Diego Rose, Ph.D., M.P.H., is Associate Professor in the Department of Community Health Sciences at the School of Public Health and Tropical Medicine, and Director of the Prevention Research Center at Tulane University. Dr. Rose holds degrees from the University of California at Berkeley in nutritional sciences (B.S.), public health nutrition (M.P.H.), and agricultural economics (Ph.D.). He began his career as a project director/nutritionist for the WIC Nutrition Program in a farm worker clinic in rural California. Dr. Rose worked for USDA's Economic Research Service as a research team leader on the determinants and consequences of household food insecurity in America, the nutrition and health impacts of food assistance programs, and the evaluation of low-income nutrition education projects. He also worked internationally on food consumption and food security projects in Mozambique and South Africa. Dr. Rose's research at Tulane focuses on the social and economic side of nutrition problems, including disparities in access to food, the links between food access and consumption, domestic and international food security, and the importance of the time dimension for U.S. nutrition policy. Currently, he has research projects funded by USDA and NCI on neighborhood access to healthy foods and its influence on consumption in New Orleans and southeast Louisiana. Dr. Rose served on the National Research Council panel to review USDA's food security measurement.

Mary T. Story, Ph.D., R.D., is Professor in the Division of Epidemiology and Community Health in the School of Public Health, University of Minnesota, Minneapolis. She is an Adjunct Professor in the Department of Pediatrics, School of Medicine at the University of Minnesota. Dr. Story has her Ph.D. in nutrition and her interests are in the area of child and adolescent nutrition, obesity prevention, and environmental and policy approaches to improve healthy eating. Her research focuses on understanding the multiple factors related to eating behaviors of youth, and environmental, community and school-based interventions for obesity prevention and healthy eating. She has over 300 journal articles and publications in the area of child and adolescent nutrition and obesity. She is the Director of the National Program Office for the Robert Wood Johnson Foundation Healthy Eating Research program. She is currently on the editorial boards for the *Journal of the American Dietetic Association*, *Journal of Adolescent Health*, and *Nutrition Today*. She has received several awards for her work. She was a member of the IOM Committee on Food Marketing to Children and Youth and the Committee on Nutrition Standards for Foods in Schools. She is a current member of the IOM Standing Committee on Childhood Obesity Prevention.

Adewale Troutman, M.D., M.P.H., M.A., is the Director of the Louisville Metro Health Department and an Associate Professor at the University of Louisville School of Public Health. He received an M.P.H. from the Columbia University School of Public Health and also earned an M.A. in Black Studies from the State University of New York. He completed medical training at the University of Medicine and Dentistry of New Jersey and served his residency and internship in Family Medicine at the Medical University of South Carolina. As Director of the Louisville Metro Health Department, Dr. Troutman created the Center for Health Equity, which focuses on eliminating health inequities based on race, ethnicity or socioeconomic status. He also established the *Mayor's Healthy Hometown*

Movement, a community wide effort to motivate the citizens of Louisville to engage in more physical activity and to adopt healthier lifestyles and the *Take Charge Challenge*, a worksite wellness program for Louisville Metro employees. Dr. Troutman has served as the Director of the Fulton County (Atlanta, Georgia) Department of Health and Wellness and as a senior scientist for Community Health and Preventive Medicine at the Morehouse School of Medicine. At Morehouse, he worked with former U.S. Surgeon General David Satcher on a study of racial disparities in health. Dr. Troutman's many leadership positions have included the Chair of the Health and Social Justice Advisory Committee of the National Association of County and City Health Officials (NACCHO), the governing board of American Public Health Association, the Presidency of the Black Caucus of Health Workers, and the Health Equity Social Justice Strategic Directors Team.

Antronette K. (Toni) Yancey, M.D., M.P.H., is Professor of Health Services and Co-Director, UCLA Kaiser Permanente Center for Health Equity at UCLA School of Public Health. She completed her B.A. in biochemistry and molecular biology at Northwestern University, her M.D. at Duke, and her preventive medicine residency and M.P.H. at UCLA. Dr. Yancey has generated over $25 million in extramural funds including four National Institutes of Health independent investigator awards as principal investigator, and authored more than 100 scientific publications, including policy briefs, reports, book chapters, radio commentaries, videos, and, among them, 75 peer-reviewed journal articles and editorials on chronic disease prevention and adolescent health, with an emphasis on urban communities of color. She spent 5 years in public health practice, as Director of Public Health for the city of Richmond, Virginia, and Director of Chronic Disease Prevention and Health Promotion for the Los Angeles County Department of Health Services. Dr. Yancey serves on the Coordinating Committee of the National Physical Activity Plan, the IOM Standing Committee on Childhood Obesity Prevention and Health Literacy Roundtable, and the editorial boards for the American Journal of Preventive Medicine and American Journal of Health Promotion. She chairs the Board of Directors of the Oakland, California-based Public Health Institute, and formerly served on the Department of Health and Human Services' Physical Activity Guidelines Advisory Committee; Board of the National Marrow Donor Program, and IOM Committee on Progress in Preventing Childhood Obesity. Her book, *Instant Recess: How to Build a Fit Nation for the 21st Century* (University of California Press), is anticipated in 2010.

Paul Zykofsky, B.Sc., BArch, M.U.P., is Director of the Land Use and Transportation Programs at the Local Government Commission (LGC) in Sacramento, California, and manages its Center for Livable Communities. He obtained the degrees of bachelor of architecture and master of urban planning from the City College of New York. Mr. Zykofsky has experience in land use, air quality, and transportation planning gained while working at a city development agency, an air quality management district and a council of governments. He is co-author of documents on transit-oriented development and street design and has edited numerous documents on sustainable development and community design. In collaboration with the California Department of Health Services, Mr. Zykofsky has directed a first-of-its-kind project to promote physical activity by improving the design of the pedestrian environment. He currently directs the LGC's Leadership for Healthy Communities project, part of a national initiative supported by The Robert Wood Johnson Foundation. Mr. Zykofsky serves on the Steering Committee of the Rail-Volution conference, an annual national conference on building livable communities with transit. He also was one of four instructors that developed and administered 3-day classes on Context Sensitive Solutions to several hundred planners and engineers in the California Department of Transportation's district offices. He facilitates workshops throughout the United States on Safe Routes to School and teaches a 2-day course for the Federal Highway Administration on designing for pedestrian safety. He also facilitates multiday design charrettes aimed at helping communities develop plans to create more walkable, bicycle-friendly places. He is a member of the American Institute of Certified Planners, an Associate Member of the American Institute of Architects and a member of the Congress for the New Urbanism. Mr. Zykofsky was born and raised in Mexico and is fluent in Spanish.

Study Staff

Lynn Parker, M.S., is a Scholar and Study Director for the Standing Committee on Childhood Obesity Prevention, the Committee on Childhood Obesity Prevention Actions for Local Governments and the Committee on an Evidence Framework for Obesity Prevention Decision Making. Ms. Parker received a B.A. in anthropology from the University of Michigan and an M.S. in human nutrition from Cornell University. Before she joined IOM, she was a nutritionist at the Food Research and Action Center (FRAC), a national organization working to end hunger and undernutrition in the United States, most recently as director of Child Nutrition Programs and Nutrition Policy, where she directed FRAC's work on child nutrition programs, research, and nutrition policy. She also led FRAC's initiative on understanding and responding to the paradox of hunger, poverty, and obesity. She served on the Technical Advisory Group to America's Second Harvest 2001 and 2005 National Hunger Surveys; the National Nutrition Monitoring Advisory Council (appointed by then Senate Majority Leader George Mitchell); and as President of the Society for Nutrition Education. She also served two terms as a member of the Food and Nutrition Board and was a member of its Committee on Nutrition Standards for Foods in Schools. Before joining FRAC, she worked with New York State's Expanded Food and Nutrition Education Program at Cornell University.

Annina Catherine Burns, M.Sc., is a Study Director for Community Perspectives on Childhood Obesity Prevention and Perspectives from United Kingdom and the United States Policymakers on Obesity Prevention. She is also Co-Study Director for Childhood Obesity Prevention: Austin, Texas. Ms. Burns previously worked for the United Nations World Health Organization (WHO) in Geneva, Switzerland, on the Global Strategy on Diet, Physical Activity and Health. At the WHO, she was a project manager and led the development of the report *Interventions on Diet and Physical Activity: What Works*. Ms. Burns was a Marshall Scholar at Oxford University, United Kingdom, where she pursued her Masters of Science in Economic and Social History and her thesis research was on *The Emergence of Obesity in Scotland: Historical and Contemporary Dietary Intakes*. She is currently completing a Ph.D. from Oxford University, with a focus on nutrition policy, obesity and economics. Ms. Burns holds a B.S. in nutritional sciences and a B.A. in media studies from Penn State University. She is the recipient of the Reddy Mission Award given to Penn State's most outstanding scholar who has integrated academic excellence, internationalization, service, and leadership.

Catharyn T. Liverman, M.L.S., is a Scholar at the IOM. In her 16 years with the IOM, she has worked on studies addressing a range of topics, focused primarily on public health and science policy. She was recently Study Director for two IOM reports on preventing childhood obesity. Other recent studies in which she was involved include *Organ Donation: Opportunities for Action*; *Spinal Cord Injury: Progress, Promise, and Priorities*; *Testosterone and Aging: Clinical Research Directions*; *Gulf War and Health*; and *Reducing the Burden of Injury*. Her background is in medical library science; she previously held positions at the National

Agricultural Library and the Naval War College Library. She received her B.A. from Wake Forest University and her M.L.S. from the University of Maryland.

Nicole Ferring, M.S., R.D., is a Research Associate with the Food and Nutrition Board. She works with the Standing Committee on Childhood Obesity Prevention and the Committee on Childhood Obesity Prevention Actions for Local Governments. Ms. Ferring previously worked for the Center for Science in the Public Interest (CSPI) on the *Nutrition Action Healthletter.* She recently finished a year-long dietetic internship through Virginia Tech to obtain the registered dietitian credential. The internship allowed her to rotate through different types of nutrition settings in the Washington, DC, area, including hospitals, community nonprofits, policy organizations, and even a farm. She holds a B.S. in magazine journalism with a minor in nutrition from Syracuse University and an M.S. in nutrition communication from Tufts University.

Matthew B. Spear, B.A., is a Senior Program Assistant with the Food and Nutrition Board. He works with the Standing Committee on Childhood Obesity Prevention, the Committee on Childhood Obesity Prevention Actions for Local Governments, and the Committee on an Evidence Framework for Obesity Prevention Decision Making. Mr. Spear holds a B.A. in economics from Boston College. He recently completed a year-long course and internship studying culinary arts in Florence, Italy, and working as a private chef. International travel and interest in languages drew him out of the kitchen and formed his interest in public policy, leading him to the IOM.

Linda D. Meyers, Ph.D., is the Food and Nutrition Board Director. Prior to assuming that position in 2003, she was Deputy Director and senior Program Officer for two years. She also directed the Food and Nutrition Board's international nutrition program from 1982 to 1986. From 1986 to 2001, she served in the Office of Disease Prevention and Health Promotion in the Department of Health and Human Services, where she was a Senior Nutrition Advisor, Deputy Director, and Acting Director. While there, she oversaw the preparation of numerous technical and policy reports, including the 1990, 1995, and 2000 *Dietary Guidelines for Americans,* the *U.S. Action Plan on Food Security,* and the national health objectives for Healthy People 2010. Dr. Meyers received a B.A. in health and physical education from Goshen College in Indiana. After 4 years in Botswana, she pursued graduate studies in nutrition at Colorado State

University (M.S. 1974) and Cornell University (Ph.D. 1978). Her research at Cornell focused on population indicators of nutritional status. Her work on the prevalence and correlates of iron deficiency anemia was among the first to identify differences in normal hemoglobin distributions between black and white women and question the use of a single hemoglobin cutpoint for prevalence estimates. Dr. Meyers has also worked in Kenya and lived in Viet Nam. She has received a number of awards for her contributions to public health, including the Secretary's Distinguished Service Award for *Healthy People 2010* and the Surgeon General's Medallion.